REVIEW MANUAL TO ACCOMPANY
HEALTH INFORMATION:
MANAGEMENT OF A STRATEGIC RESOURCE

Beverli H. Reding, PhD, RRA
Mary Alice Hanken, PhD, RRA

Managing Editor
MERVAT ABDELHAK, PhD, RRA

Chairman, Health Information Management Department
  and Associate Professor
School of Health & Rehabilitative Sciences
University of Pittsburgh
Pittsburgh, PA

Editors
SARA GROSTICK, MA, RRA

Director, Health Information Management Program
  and Associate Professor
School of Health Related Professions
University of Alabama in Birmingham
Birmingham, AL

MARY ALICE HANKEN, PhD, RRA

Director, Health Information Administration Program
School of Public Health and Community Medicine
University of Washington
Seattle, WA

ELLEN JACOBS, MEd, RRA

Director and Associate Professor,
  Health Information Management Program
College of St. Mary
Omaha, NE

W.B. SAUNDERS COMPANY

A Division of Harcourt Brace & Company
Philadelphia   London   Toronto
Montreal   Sydney   Tokyo

W. B. Saunders Company
A Division of Harcourt Brace & Company
The Curtis Center
Independence Square West
Philadelphia, PA 19106

Review Manual to Accompany
HEALTH INFORMATION: Management of a Strategic Resource

ISBN 0-7216-5148-8

Printed in the United States of America

Last digit is the print number: 9   8   7   6   5   4   3   2

CONTENTS

PREFACE

This review manual is created to benefit students preparing for course and unit examinations, practitioners working toward continuing education credits, and graduates facing the certification examination. Practitioners may also find it useful for inservice education, pre-employment and employment training. It is made up of 1000 questions with answers for each chapter, except Chapter 19, in the companion book— *Health Information: Management of a Strategic Resource.* Each chapter in this review manual includes pretests, comprehensive reviews, and performance grids for charting scores.While these are only a sampling of all possible questions on each subject, they will provide some immediate feedback on how well you are understanding and beginning to apply the material you are learning if you are in a student-learning mode.

It is important to read Section One - How to Use This Review Manual— before attempting to answer the questions. This section explains how the book is constructed and how to get the most out of it.

All the questions in Section Two, which measure your understanding and application of the chapter objectives, are written by outstanding educators and practitioners. Section Three explains the certification exam and how to prepare for it.

I would like to take this opportunity to express my sincere appreciation to all the contributors, and to their many colleagues, who were also thoughtfully committed to this first edition. It is hoped by all of us that this review manual will facilitate your mastery of each subject and will attempt to pull all the subjects together as you proceed chapter-by-chapter. We wish you well in your personal effort.

Beverli H. Reding, PhD, RRA
Consultant

CONTRIBUTING AUTHORS

Carol J. Barr, MA, RRA
Director, Health Information Management Program, University of Central Florida, Orlando, Florida
Human Resources Management

Elizabeth D. Bowman, MPA, RRA
Associate Professor, Department of Health Information Management, The University of Tennessee, Memphis, Tennessee
Coding and Classification Systems

Jill Callahan Dennis, JD, RRA
Principal, Health Risk Advantage, Winfield, Illinois
Health Law Concepts and Practices

W. Jack Duncan, MBA, PhD
Professor and University Scholar, Graduate School of Management. Professor of Health Care Organization, School of Public Health, University of Alabama at Birmingham, Birmingham, Alabama
Principles of Management

Rose T. Dunn, MBA, RRA, CPA, FACHE
Vice President, First Class Solutions, Inc., St. Louis, Missouri
Financial Management

Peter M. Ginter, MBA, PhD
Professor, Graduate School of Management. Professor, Health Care Organization and Policy, School of Public Health, University of Alabama at Birmingham, Birmingham, Alabama
Principles of Management

Merida L. Johns, PhD, RRA
Associate Professor and Director, Master of Science in Health Information Management, University of Alabama at Birmingham, Birmingham, Alabama
Information Systems Life Cycle

Lynn Kuehn, MS, RRA
Operations Administrator, Family Health Systems, Milwaukee, Wisconsin
Data Access and Retention

Jeanette C. Linck, MA, MPA, RRA
Central Office Coordinator, Michigan Health Information Management Association, Ravenna, Michigan
Patient and Health Care Data

Gretchen F. Murphy, MEd, RRA
Senior Project Manager, Group Health Cooperative. Lecturer, Health Information Administration, Department of Health Sciences, School of Public Health and Community Medicine, University of Washington, Seattle, Washington
Computer-Based Patient Records: A Unifying Principle

Midge Noel Ray, RN, MSN
Associate Professor, Health Information Management Program, Department of Health Services Administration, School of Health-Related Professions, University of Alabama at Birmingham, Birmingham, Alabama
Health Care Systems

Wesley M. Rohrer III, MBA, PhD
Assistent Professor, Department of Health Information Management, and Associate Dean, School of Health and Rehabilitation Sciences, University of Pittsburgh, Pittsburgh, Pennsylvania
Human Relations

William J. Rudman, PhD
Associate Professor, School of Health Related Professions (Medical Center), University of Mississippi, Jackson, Mississippi
Human Relations

Rita A. Scichilone, MHSA, RRA, CCS
Adjunct Faculty, College of St. Mary. Health Information Program. Consultant, Reimbursement Specialist; Professional Management Midwest, Omaha, Nebraska
Human Resources Management

Donna J. Slovensky, MA, RRA
Associate Professor, Department of Health Services Administration, School of Health Related Professions, University of Alabama at Birmingham, Birmingham, Alabama
Quality Assessment and Improvement

Mary Spivey, MLIS, RRA
Program Coordinator, Health Information Management, Broward Community College, Fort Lauderdale, Florida
Data Collection

Mildred P. St. Leger, BA, RRA
Assistent Professor and Director, Health Information Management, College of Health Sciences, Roanoke, Virginia
The Health Information Management Profession

Sue Watkins, AS, ART, CTR
Director, Tri-Counties Regional Cancer Registry and Health Information Services, Santa Barbara County Health Care Services, Santa Barbara, California
Registries

Valerie J.M. Watzlaf, PhD, RRA
Assistant Professor, Department of Health Information Management, School of Health and Rehabilitation Sciences, University of Pittsburgh. Pittsburgh, Pennsylvania
Research, Statistics, and Epidemiology

Donna J. Wilde, MPA, RRA
Professor, Health Care Information Programs, Shoreline Community College, Seattle, Washington
Data Quality

Karen G. Youmans, MPA, RRA, CCS
Instructor, Health Information Management Program, University of Central Florida, Orlando, Florida
Methods for Analyzing and Improving Systems

SECTION ONE

How to Use this Review Manual

PURPOSES OF REVIEW MANUAL

The principal purpose of this review manual is the self-examination of your mastery of the subject matter in the accompanying book. Since answers are provided for each question in answer keys, you can determine subject areas of weakness and return to the book for further study. Key terms and principles are noted in bold type throughout the chapters in the book enabling rapid location and reference for this purpose.

The intent of this review manual is not to memorize questions and answers, thinking that they may be repeated on an actual examination, but rather to assess and reinforce your understanding of theories, principles, concepts, and terms, including related information, so that you can be successful in answering any question on that subject correctly. This ability comes with careful reading and rereading of the book and collateral references, and not in becoming question dependent.

In addition to the principal purpose, additional purposes can be realized. This comprehensive review approach can also enhance your performance of certain tasks and your solving of simulated problems. Other purposes of the *Review Manual to Accompany Health Information: Management of a Strategic Resource* include:

- Increase your confidence
- Measure unit examination readiness by chapter
- Enable testing experience
- Provide opportunity for last-minute review
- Supply repeated review opportunities
- Increase practice skills in certain tasks and subtasks
- Expand your knowledge and/or competence base

While the remaining sections in this Introduction are primarily for students, health information practitoners may also gain considerable insight into mastery preparation by reviewing the information that is supplied.

HELPFUL STUDY TECHNIQUES

Before attempting to use this review manual, evaluate your approach to studying. Is your study plan working for you or can it be improved? The following discussion may assist in refining your approach to studying.

BASIC STUDY TECHNIQUES

1. **Scan all your learning resources for a unit.**

Survey the chapter, paying attention to headings, subheadings, topic sentences and summaries. Include your exercise book, handouts, notes and this review manual (corresponding also to the learning unit in progress). When you get a broad view of the whole, the parts take on added meaning — how they all fit together. This helps to eliminate surprises and to give you a feeling for the breadth of the task.

2. **Study the objectives for each chapter.**

Focus on the verb. Are you expected to define, list, describe or recognize? Whatever the verb used, it will suggest how you may be tested. Short essay questions requiring a one-sentence response may be used to define terms; matching questions to identify definitions, principles or concepts. Regular essay questions may be used for asking your description of a broader concept or principle, or your justification for a response, such as can be answered in one or more brief paragraphs. Short completion questions may be used when the objective asks you to list, name or identify something. The types of questions to be used in this review manual are discussed elsewhere in this section.

Always write out answers to objectives and be sure to be guided by any additional objectives supplied by your instructor; verify with your instructor all the chapter objectives for which you are responsible. Answering objectives can be done concurrently with reading the chapter, for the process can enhance your comprehension of the material.

3. **Read the entire textbook chapter, including key terms.**

Glance over the chapter outline, chapter objectives and key terms before proceeding in reading to determine the important subject matter requiring significant attention. This review manual emphasizes that foundational content, particularly the objectives. (Note: Reading is a most important phase of learning that requires the highest level of concentration. Any outside noise can subconsciously be distracting thereby negatively impacting your concentration without one consciously realizing it. Attempt to find the quietest place for this exercise.)

4. **Underscore or highlight principles, theories, purposes, rationales and basic concepts that correspond with the objectives.**

This process emphasizes their learning in the context in which they have been written in the text.

5. Develop mini outlines of a principle or related principles that appear over the course of several pages in the textbook.

Use 3 x 5 cards or regular notebook paper if it would facilitate storage. For example, chapter objective 3-3 states: "Identify and define characteristics of data quality." As you are reading the chapter you discover that these nine (9) characteristics of data quality are discussed over 2-3 pages: validity, reliability, completeness, legibility, timeliness, usefulness, accessibility, confidentiality and legality. From this, your mini-outline can illustrate the fundamental information, and by alphabetizing the characteristics, facilitate easier recall of the information in its total context:

Mini-Outline

Objective 3-3:
Characteristics of data quality - meaning data has quality when it is:

1. accessible
2. complete
3. confidential & secure
4. current and timely
5. legal
6. legible
7. meaningful & useful
8. reliable
9. valid

(Note: See key terms for definitions)

Since definitions are provided for these terms in the Glossary of the text, little may be gained by writing out the definitions. A note to yourself on this point is added to the mini-outline.

6. Organize all your learning materials.

Get them all together for each chapter: answers to objectives, lecture notes, lab exercises and handouts. (Note: Some students assemble all materials from all sources in a 3-ring notebook for each subject unit. Upon preparing for finals and the certification examination, they simply review the same material in the order they learned it originally without any additional organization required).

7. Begin your review early.

Review is designed to assist in recall; it cannot be accomplished hastily. Even if you recall information easily, review in order to "over learn." It builds confidence, reduces anxiety, and should translate into correct application.

HELPFUL TEST-TAKING PRINCIPLES

In addition to subject preparation, taking and passing examinations is dependent upon other factors also. The following principles are general and not necessarily unique and applicable only to this review manual or subject matter. These principles are suggested to act as guidelines, and not absolutes, in choosing the best response for a question.

1. **Find out how the test is scored.** This may be stated in the test directions, in the course syllabus, or in pre-printed test materials. Be sure that guessing or failing to answer all the questions will not hurt your score. Knowing the scoring methodology enables you to set your test-writing strategy in advance.

2. **Find out the types of questions to be asked.** Again, this is important in developing your studying strategy. If the test is all essay, your study approach may be different than if it were all multiple choice.

3. **Become familiar with the types of questions.** In this review manual, six types of questions are used.

> **Multiple Choice Questions**—A question is asked in a stem followed by 1 correct or best answer and 3 distracters or wrong answers. Oftentimes, a distracter may be partially correct, in which case, it is not the best answer. Be sure to compare all four or five alternative choices against the stem of the question— not to each other—before making your choice.

Examples:

Which is a person who acts as an intermediary between someone needing data (customer), and the data sources (supplier), by providing required information?

a. data entry operator
b. data broker
c. data query engineer
d. data technician

Answer: b

Which is a research study design that deals only with survivors; is not effective in studying rare diseases; and will often miss an epidemic?

a. case-control study
b. prospective study
c. cross-sectional study
d. clinical trial

Answer: c

True/False Questions—This type of question asks if a statement is true. The entire statement must be true to denote true, otherwise, it is not true, but is false. Determine the correct answer only by the information stated; do not attempt to read into the question information that is not there.

Examples:

The current title of the national organization of Accredited Record Technicians (ARTs) and Registered Record Administrators (RRAs) is the American Medical Record Association.

a. True
b. False

Answer: b

An executive information system is a type of decision support system.

a. True
b. False

Answer: b

Yes/No Question —This type of question asks your agreement or opinion about information. If your agreement is yes, select yes; if your agreement is no, select no.

Examples:

A student in a health care professional training program enters the HIM department and asks for Mr. Rocky State's most recent health record. Since the student is on clinical experience, she should be permitted access to Mr. State's patient record. Do you agree?

a. Yes
b. No

Answer: b

Your human resources director is urging you to develop a transcriptionist training program. She has argued that there is no capital investment involved in the development of the new service because you already have dictation and transcription equipment. Do you agree that this is an accurate statement?

a. Yes
b. No

Answer: b

Problem Solving Questions—A question provides a scenario or brief write-up of an incident, situation or problem followed by one or more questions. To answer questions correctly you need to analyze multiple facts in the scenario and draw on multiple understandings of related information in your mind in order to form a correct or best response. Sometimes, extraneous information is included in the statement that is not needed for solving the problem; select out unrelated information by marking through it.

Examples:

Cafe Latte Medical Center has an average of 988 discharges per month and 341 operations. They have 183 delinquent records. They have 17 missing history and physicals. They have two Type I deficiencies.

a. True
b. False

Answer: b

A year ago a skilled nursing facility purchased a computer system to process billing claims. Six months ago, the administrative office also acquired a computer system to support clerical functions. Two months ago a system was purchased to assist with dietary planning.

Referring to the information above, which of the following stages of Nolan's Information Life Cycle is this organization likely at?

a.   initiation
b.   expansion
c.   control
d.   integration

Answer: b

Short Answer Questions—This type of question requires a one-or-more word answer and not a complete statement, such as a sentence or brief paragraph. It is used to measure the recall of simple facts, terms, abbreviations or symbols. Oftentimes, a term is asked for to complete a statement or sentence. You may also be asked to name or interpret diagrams, charts or tables from given illustrations using this question type.

Examples:

In your facility's patient database, you have a column for *date of discharge*. Give one of many edits you can build into the computer system to help the data entry operator input that data item correctly.

Answer: must be in MM//DD/YYYY format; may not be blank (other possibilities not mentioned here)

A _____ chart is a scheduling device that is a system of diagramming steps or component parts of a complex project.

Answer: PERT

Referring to the following figure, what statistical measure can be best illustrated using this type of diagram?

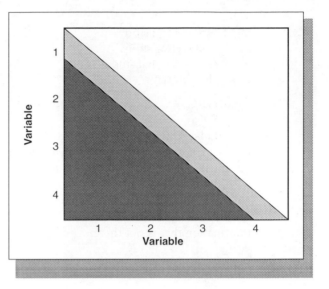

Answer: Correlation coefficient

Matching Questions—This question asks the respondent to associate terms or brief statements in one column with correct descripters of those statements in another column. In this question type, the answer is provided. Work within one column at a time, more easily the lefthand column, matching each term to the best statement in the column on the right. Place a thin pencil line through items on the right that are matched so that they will not interfere with subsequent matching. Match each item carefully, because if you change one, it may mean changing three or more. After you have marked all of the responses you are certain about, complete the matching by guessing on remaining items. (Note: Oftentimes, additional items will be provided in one or both columns for which a correct or best answer is not provided.)

Example:

Match the items in the left column with the correct descriptor in the right column. Some descriptors may not have answers.

_____ 1. database

_____ 2. data file

_____ 3. data dictionary

_____ 4. data label

_____ 5. data steward

_____ 6. data type

a. alpha or numeric

b. smallest unit of data

c. Describe objects related to a data element

d. information about stored data

e. protects databases

f. stores data

g. data name

h. data table

Answers: 1. f   4. g

2. h   5. e

3. d   6. a

(Note: While essay questions are not utilized in this review manual, they are a type of question which are frequently used in test measurement to assess learning at more complex levels. For this reason, a reference is made to this type of question in the event a user of this review manual may be faced with organizing a response to an essay question).

Essay Questions—This type of question requires a one or more paragraph response. The intent is to measure one's ability to form an accurate, yet cohesive, logical and concise statement that another person could understand - much like speaking to another person. It is suggested that on the back of the test copy you pencil a brief outline of the key points you intend to discuss; order the points by number and then formulate your response from the outline. This prevents you from accidently dropping from the answer process a key

point while discussing another. Write clearly, concisely and directly to the question only.

Example:

Discuss the purpose of health records.

Answer: There are several purposes the health record serves; these mentioned are but a few. The principal purpose is to provide a historical record for the patient that will serve as a foundation for continued quality care in the future. Second, the health record is maintained as a legal document for the benefit of the patient and the provider(s). Third, the health record serves as a basis for evaluating and improving the quality of care; for planning; for research, and for remuneration of patient services.

4. **Bring to every test at least two pencils and a calculator.** Paper and notes are not generally allowed so that any calculations will have to be noted on the back of your answer sheet or in the test booklet. It is recommended that you provide yourself with an audit trail by making notes of all your math in the event you make an incorrect choice. (Note: Calculators and table surfaces may be examined by a circulating test proctor, periodically.0

5. **Read the directions for the test carefully and listen intently to any oral instructions given.** Generally, once an examination begins, there will be no questions answered. If you do not understand something in the directions, be sure to speak up and ask right away.

6. **Study the answer sheet carefully and keep checking it throughout the test to make certain you are filling in the answer sheet for the question you intend to answer.** Sometimes a question number is skipped because the student intended to come back to it. Be sure to flag those questions in some way *on the answer sheet* so as not to inadvertently record the answer to the next successive question in its spot. Generally, answer sheets are graded by machine. Care should be given to shade in your answer completely as noted and to erase completely, as shown:

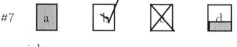

right way   wrong ways

7. **Pace yourself by wearing a watch or sitting in view of a clock.** To prepare for this, flip through all the pages of the test before beginning to obtain an overview of its scope and layout. Familiarizing yourself with what is ahead, rather than waiting to be surprised when it may be too late, will enable you to plan your time for certain sections of the examination rather than react to a lack of sufficient time.

   Many tests are not timed, but if they are, remember that the scoring may be calculated on the percent of questions you answered correctly out of the total you attempted. This means that questions you did not have time to get to will not affect your score.

8. **Be clear about what each question is asking before attempting a response.** Reread each question and underscore key words to ensure clarity. (Note: Did you miss any of the examples above because you misread the question?)

9. **Read each possible answer before marking your choice.** Many questions may contain two or more very similar answers from which you must choose the best or most correct answer. If you have trouble in selecting a correct or best answer, skip the question. Perhaps information within subsequent questions will trigger a correct response in your mind or provide contributing information for selecting a correct answer; **be certain** to mark the question you are skipping on your answer sheet as a reminder to return to it.

10. **Before finishing an examination section, or the complete exam, go over it thoroughly to be certain all answers have been recorded.**

PREPARING FOR CHAPTER REVIEWS

Review questions are provided for Chapters 1-18. For each chapter there are a total of 60 questions, 12 of which have been organized into a Pretest Review. Subsequent to each Pretest Review is a more comprehensive review for each chapter comprised of 48 questions called a Chapter Review. All questions are based on the accompanying textbook—*Health Information: Management of A Strategic Resource.*

This review manual presupposes that you have already learned these subjects:

- Anatomy and Physiology
- Medical Terminology
- Medical Science
- Coding Practice Skills

A wide range of topics are covered in this review manual. Topics not discussed in the textbook are also not included in this review manual. Some questions test your knowledge or recall of fundamental information and principles, while others require you to apply information, principles, standards or theory to a problem situation. Consequently, the level of difficulty increases as the nature of the question moves from a recall-type question to an application or problem-solving type. The time required to answer application and problem-solving type questions also increases from that required of recall-type questions. This should be taken into consideration when scheduling your time on actual examinations; the time to complete certain review questions in this manual can serve as a benchmark for this purpose.

PRETEST REVIEWS

Each Pretest Review enables a quick self-assessment of factual knowledge pertaining to the chapter. This is accomplished by the use of true/false-type questions. Use the pretest review after the initial reading of the chapter, preferably before pursuing any application exercises of the material. At the end of each chapter in this review manual is a Pretest Review Answer Key for correcting your answers. Although brief, the Pretest Review will help to alert you to any misunderstandings or principles not yet fully comprehended before you attempt the more comprehensive Chapter Review.

CHAPTER REVIEWS

Following each Pretest Review are 48 Chapter Review questions utilizing the six types of questions discussed previously. Its purpose is to measure your pre-examination readiness of the chapter subject matter. The intent is to complete the Chapter Review during the process of overall examination preparation and to correct your responses promptly using the Chapter Review Answer Key located at the back of each chapter.

The results of your performance may necessitate further study of selected portions of the textbook and of lecture notes. To assist you in interpreting your performance, a Performance Grid is provided.

PREPARING PERFORMANCE GRIDS

In Section Four there are three Performance Grids for you to chart your overall test performance and mastery of the textbook subject material chapter-by-chapter. The Initial Performance Grid (found in the last section of this review manual) is needed for the first-time completion of this review book. The Repeat Performance Grids may be used for subsequent reviews at your own discretion, particularly if you are a student preparing for final examinations and your certification examination.

For example, assume you have just completed a Pretest Review for Chapter l in the textbook. You missed two questions. You record the remaining 10 which are correct in Column 2. To calculate the percent of correct responses for this Pretest Review, simply divide the number 10 by the total correct responses possible, which was 12, and record the percent in Column 3. You demonstrated a correct understanding of 83% of the subject matter.

Since this Pretest Review sample is small, it should be used only as an indication of readiness to proceed with the Chapter Review. Be sure to study the correct answers for all answers missed in the respective chapter of the text; restudy the context of the subject matter surrounding that which pertained to the questions you missed. Since your overall performance on this Pretest Review was greater than 80%, and you have restudied your areas of weakness, you decide to proceed to the Chapter Review.

Assume now that you have just completed the Chapter Review. Upon correcting your Chapter Review Test with the Answer Key at the back of the chapter, you missed 13. You subtract the 13 wrong from the total questions in the Chapter Review which was 48 to obtain the total number of questions you answered correctly. Record 35 correct answers in Column 5 and proceed to calculate the percent correct as you did for the Pretest Review, above. Record 73% in Column 6 on the Initial Performance Grid.

You demonstrated 73% understanding of the content of the Chapter Review. Since this is less than 75%, which is considered passing by some standards, again you should reread those portions of the chapter where the principles are discussed for each question missed. In this instance, finding out why you missed each question by simply examining a page in the textbook may be insufficient for fully grasping the material; rereading the subject matter in the broader context surrounding that which pertained to the questions missed is the recommended solution for improving your mastery.

You may want to aim at an 80% or higher mastery performance overall. It depends on the grading standards for your coursework. In this example, the student's overall chapter mastery—the Pretest Review performance plus the Chapter Review performance—was calculated to be 75%. This was obtained by summing the number correct on the Pretest Review from Column 2 with the number correct on the Chapter Review in Column 5 and dividing that sum by the total number of questions in both review tests which is 60 (Column 1 + Column 4). This overall percent is recorded in Column 7. Aiming for a higher mastery than needed to pass a unit test or a final examination helps to establish a margin for error due to carelessness, misreading or some other reason. Aiming at 100% mastery is not an unreasonable review goal. Consider it an opportunity.

WORKING WITH CRITICAL COMPETENCE QUESTIONS

Many of the questions in this manual may be representative of the questions which will be used in unit and final examinations by college and university health information management programs. While the content of the questions may also be representative of that tested in the national certifying examinations (discussed in Section Three—How to Prepare for Certification), the question type will be different. Ordinarily, the certifying examinations utilize only multiple choice-type questions and not the variety that is used here or in some colleges and universities for teaching purposes.

Since subject content and its mastery is prerequisite to competent performance as a certified practitioner, this review manual includes for your reference the *Entry-level Competencies for Accredited Record Technicians and Registered Record Administrators* on the succeeding pages. These statements form the basis for certification examination test construction. Notice the "knowledges" explicated in order to be able to perform the designated tasks and subtasks. Examination questions in this review manual also emphasize these stated, essential knowledges. So, be familiar with the "knowledges" required for your respective entrance level competence—Accredited Record Technician or Registered Record Administrator—and incorporate them into your personal review process. Most education programs distribute the current list of competencies to students for reference throughout their coursework. When graduates make application for the certification examination, the test materials mailed to the applicant contain a current list of the competencies to be tested.

AMERICAN HEALTH INFORMATION MANAGEMENT ASSOCIATION

Domains, Tasks, and Subtasks

(Entry Level Competencies)

for Accredited Record Technicians

Domains, Tasks, and Subtasks

Domain 1

Assess institutional and patient-related information needs and departmental, (i.e., medical record, quality assurance, cancer registry, or similar department) informational, service, and operational needs.

Task

1.1 Gather data to support patient-related information system needs and departmental operations and services.

Subtasks

1.1.1 Conduct surveys of patients, users of data, healthcare providers, administrators, and/or researchers.

1.1.2 Conduct interviews with users of data, healthcare providers, administrators, researchers, and/or others.

1.1.3 Tabulate requests for patient-related data.

1.1.4 Monitor changes in federal, state, and local laws, regulations, and/or Joint Commission standards.

1.1.5 Monitor departmental productivity.

1.1.6 Collect data on employee performance.

1.1.7 Compare claims submitted to third-party payers with reimbursement received.

1.1.8 Monitor work flow under your span of control.

1.1.9 Collect data on the quality of documentation in the medical record (i.e., timeliness, completeness, accuracy).

1.1.10 Tabulate data on the appropriateness and quality of patient care as documented in the medical record (i.e., quality assurance, utilization review activities).

1.1.11 Collect data on the status of incomplete records.

1.1.12 Track location of medical records.

1.1.13 Monitor employee staffing levels.

1.1.14 Monitor accreditation/licensing survey results (i.e., Joint Commission, Medicare, etc.).

1.1.15 Monitor the release of information to ensure confidentiality of patient-related data.

1.1.16 Abstract information from patient records (concurrently or retrospectively) for quality assurance studies, utilization review, risk management.

1.1.17 Assemble medical records.

1.1.18 Release patient-related data (i.e., for reimbursement, research, legal, or patient-care related purposes).

1.1.19 Design forms for collection of patient-related and/or other data (i.e., medical record forms, quality assurance, utilization review forms, etc.).

1.1.20 Abstract information from patient records (concurrently or retrospectively) for research studies.

1.1.21 Abstract information from patient records (concurrently or retrospectively) for reimbursement.

1.1.22 Abstract information from patient records (concurrently or retrospectively) for disease, procedure, physician, or other indices.

1.1.23 Abstract information from patient records (concurrently or retrospectively) for compilation or registries.

1.1.24 Abstract information from patient records (concurrently or retrospectively) for compilation of vital statistics.

1.1.25 Abstract information from patient-related records (concurrently or retrospectively) to develop user (i.e., physician) profiles.

1.1.26 Confer with peers, providers, and/or users of departmental or institutional services.

1.1.27 Retrieve and/or file records.

1.1.28 Perform concurrent medical record review.

1.1.29 Participate in departmental and/or institutional committees.

1.1.30 Assign severity of illness categories.

1.1.31 Assign diagnostic/procedure codes using ICD-9-CM, CPT, HCPCS, DSM, or other coding systems.

Knowledge of:

K-1 Accreditation standards related to patient-related data (accreditation standards for various types of facilities)

K-2 Federal and state regulations related to patient-related data (regulations for various types of facilities)

K-5 Work measurement and analysis

K-6   Professional practice standards (i.e., AHIMA and other related data regulations for various types of facilities)

K-8   Disease process

K-9   Language of medicine (i.e., medical terminology)

K-12 Legal requirements for confidentiality of patient-related data (federal and state)

K-13 Medical record content

K-14 Record/information control system

K-15 Vital statistics (i.e., state and federal regulations, and procedures for collection and reporting)

K-16 Communication techniques (oral: interpersonal, small group, professional speaking; written: business and professional writing)

K-17 Record filing systems

K-18 Healthcare facility organization

K-19 Healthcare facility committees (i.e., medical staff, administrative including Medical Record, Quality Assurance, Risk Management, etc.)

K-20 Business/committee procedures and rules of order

K-21 Case-mix systems (i.e., DRGs, APACHE, Medisgroups, etc.)

K-22 Medical nomenclatures and diagnostic classification systems (i.e., ICD-9-CM, CPT, HCPCS, DSM, etc.)

K-48 Cancer staging systems

Skill at:

S-1   Survey instrument design (i.e., written and interview)

S-2   Interviewing

S-5   Work measurement techniques

S-7   Data presentation (manual and computer)

S-8   Data collection techniques

S-9   Data analysis

S-10 Interpretation of medical record content

S-12 Collection and compilation of vital statistics

S-13 Interpersonal and small group communications

S-14 Filing procedures (i.e., alphabetical, numerical)

S-17 Applying principles of diagnostic classification systems

S-18 Apply case-mix algorithms

S-28 Cancer staging

Task

1.2   Validate data for patient-related information systems needs, or for departmental operations or services.

Subtasks

1.2.1 Verify that data have been obtained from valid sources.

1.2.2 Verify timeliness, completeness, accuracy, and appropriateness of data sources (patient care, management, billing reports, and/or databases).

1.2.3 Compare data with standards (i.e., length of stay norms, Medicare mortality rates, departmental productivity standards, etc.).

1.2.4 Check data for internal consistency.

1.2.5 Perform edit checks to monitor data accuracy.

1.2.6 Compare data with other data sources/references to determine consistency.

1.2.7 Validate diagnostic and procedure coding (i.e., ICD-9-CM, CPT, HCPCS, or other coding systems).

1.2.8 Validate DRG assignment.

1.2.9 Validate output on UB-82 or other billing forms.

Knowledge of:

K-1; K-2; K-7 - K-9; K-13 - K-15; K-19; K-21; K-22

K-23 Data verification techniques

K-24 Peer review organization standards/procedures

Skill at:

S-6   Quality control methods

S-9   **Data analysis**

S-10; S-17 - S-18

S-19 Critical thinking

Task

1.3   Analyze data for patient-related information system needs or for departmental operations or services.

Subtasks

1.3.1 Prepare data for analysis (i.e., compile data, develop graphs, tables, etc.).

1.3.2 Perform departmental/institutional case-mix analysis.

1.3.3 Analyze patient care/institutional data in relation to regulatory and accreditation standards.

1.3.4 Analyze employee performance data in relation to departmental/institutional performance standards.

1.3.5 Calculate institutional statistics (i.e., occupancy rates, census, length of stay).

1.3.6 Analyze case-mix payment rates (i.e., DRG and others) to determine reimbursement optimization.

Knowledge of:

K-1; K-2; K-5 - K-9; K-13; K-15; K-18 - K-22

K-24 Peer review organization standards/procedures

K-25 Statistical techniques

K-26 Data presentation techniques

K-28 Computer statistical packages (i.e., SPSS, SAS, etc.)

K-29 Principles/methods for assessing patient care quality and effectiveness

K-30 Principles/methods for resources for patient care

K-31 Principles/methods of risk management

Skill at:

S-1; S-5; S-7 - S-10; S-18; S-19

S-20 Applying procedures for assessing patient care quality/effectiveness

S-21 Interpretation of statistical data.

Domains, Tasks, and Subtasks

Domain 2

Design and select departmental service and operational systems, and information systems for patient-related data.

Task

2.1 Design departmental service and operational systems.

Subtasks

2.1.1 Develop departmental plans, goals, and objectives for areas under your span of control.

2.1.2 Develop/revise departmental policies.

2.1.3 Develop/revise departmental procedures.

2.1.4 Develop/revise job descriptions.

2.1.5 Develop transition plans for implementation of new or revised systems.

2.1.6 Develop goals and objectives for computerized information systems (i.e., department or other facility systems).

2.1.7 Develop inservice education programs for departmental or non-departmental staff.

Knowledge of:

K-1 - K-7; K-10 - K-15; K-17 - K-19; K-21 - K-25; K-30; K-31

K-32 Management principles of planning and organizing

K-33 Functions related to Medical Record, Utilization Management, Quality Assurance, Cancer Registry, and related departments

K-34 Management principles of controlling

K-35 Business and professional writing techniques

K-36 Principles of job analysis

K-37 General systems principles

K-38 Work simplification techniques

K-39 Forms design and management

K-40 Information technologies

K-41 Systems analysis design, development, and implementation principles

K-42 Project planning

K-43 Data security techniques (manual and computer)

K-44 Space management

K-49 Principles of inservice education

Skill at:

S-6; S-8; S-9; S-11; S-19 - S-21

S-22 Professional and business writing

S-23 Applying work simplification techniques

S-24 Systems analysis

S-25 Applying project planning techniques

S-26 Inservice education development/presentation

Task

2.2 Identify/select resources to support departmental operations and information systems.

Subtasks

2.2.1 Determine personnel needs for staffing current and/or new systems.

2.2.2 Determine equipment and/or supply needs for current and/or new systems.

2.2.3 Determine space requirements for current and/or new systems.

Knowledge of:

K-5; K-10; K-17; K-33; K-36; K-40

K-45 Methods/procedures for procurement, maintenance, and selection of equipment and supplies.

Skill at:

S-9; S-19; S-21; S-23

Domains, Tasks, and Subtasks

Domain 3

Implement departmental service and operational systems, and information systems for patient-related data.

Task

3.1   Execute plan(s) for implementing departmental service and operational systems, and information systems for patient-related data.

Subtasks

3.1.1   Select personnel.

3.1.2   Train personnel.

3.1.3   Inform organization staff of plan(s).

3.1.4   Implement new-revised policies and procedures.

3.1.5   Monitor adherence to system specifications.

3.1.6   Implement new-revised information, and/or service, and/or operational systems.

3.1.7   Monitor adherence to budget (i.e., determine budget variance, etc.).

3.1.8   Coordinate on-site review activities (i.e., PRO reviews, etc.).

3.1.9   Monitor policy/procedure compliance.

3.1.10   Counsel/discipline employees.

3.1.11   Terminate employees.

3.1.12   Design employee staffing schedules.

3.1.13   Maintain equipment (i.e., schedule preventive maintenance, arrange for repairs, etc.).

3.1.14   Educate medical record and/or other students assigned to the facility.

3.1.15   Conduct educational programs for departmental and/or non-departmental staff.

Knowledge of:

K-3 - K-5; K-16; K-18; K-32; K-33; K-34; K-35; K-45

K-46   Principles of human resources management

K-47   Principles of organizational behavior

K-49   Inservice education design and presentation

Skill at:

S-2; S-3; S-5; S-6; S-9; S-11; S-19; S-21; S-25;

S-27   Applying principles of human resources management (i.e., selecting, training, motivating, promoting personnel, etc.)

Domains, Tasks, and Subtasks

Domain 4

Evaluate departmental, operational and service systems, and information systems for patient-related data.

Task

4.1   Evaluate the effectiveness and efficiency of departmental, operational and service systems, and information systems for patient-related data.

Subtasks

4.1.1   Determine variation(s) from established objectives and/or standards of performance.

4.1.2   Recommend changes and/or improvement(s) in systems.

4.1.3   Evaluate employee performance.

Knowledge of:

K-1; K-2; K-6 - K-7; K-11 - K-17; K-19; K-21 - K-25; K-28 - K-40; K-43 - K-47

Skill at:

S-1 -S-2; S-5 - S-6; S-8; S-9; S-19; S-20 - S-22; S-27

AMERICAN HEALTH INFORMATION MANAGEMENT ASSOCIATION

Domains, Tasks, and Subtasks

(Entry Level Competencies)

for Registered Record Administrators

Domains, Tasks, and Subtasks

Domain 1

Assess institutional and patient-related information needs and departmental, (i.e., medical record, quality assurance, cancer registry, or similar department) informational, service, and operational needs.

Tasks

1.1 Gather data to support patient-related information system needs and departmental operations and services.

Subtasks

1.1.1 Conduct surveys of patients, users of data, healthcare providers, administrators, and/or researchers.

1.1.2 Conduct interviews with users of data, healthcare providers, administrators, researchers, and/or others.

1.1.3 Tabulate requests for patient-related data.

1.1.4 Monitor changes in federal, state, and local laws, regulations, and/or Joint Commission standards.

1.1.5 Monitor departmental productivity.

1.1.6 Collect data on employee performance.

1.1.7 Compare claims submitted to third-party payers with reimbursement received.

1.1.8 Monitor work flow under your span of control.

1.1.9 Collect data on the quality of documentation in the medical record (i.e., timeliness, completeness, accuracy).

1.1.10 Tabulate data on the appropriateness and quality of patient care as documented in the medical record (i.e., quality assurance, utilization review activities).

1.1.11 Collect data on the status of incomplete records.

1.1.12 Track location of medical records.

1.1.13 Monitor employee staffing levels.

1.1.14 Monitor accreditation/licensing survey results (i.e., Joint Commission, Medicare, etc.).

1.1.15 Monitor the release of information to ensure confidentiality of patient-related data.

1.1.16 Abstract information from patient records (concurrently or retrospectively) for quality assurance studies, utilization review, risk management.

1.1.17 Release patient-related data (i.e., for reimbursement, research, legal, or patient-care related purposes).

1.1.18 Design forms for collection of patient-related and/or other data (i.e., medical record forms, quality assurance, utilization review forms, etc.).

1.1.19 Abstract information from patient records (concurrently or retrospectively) for research studies.

1.1.20 Abstract information from patient records (concurrently or retrospectively) for reimbursement.

1.1.21 Abstract information from patient records (concurrently or retrospectively) for disease, procedure, physician, or other indices.

1.1.22 Abstract information from patient records (concurrently or retrospectively) for compilation of registries.

1.1.23 Abstract information from patient records (concurrently or retrospectively) for compilation for vital statistics.

1.1.24 Abstract information from patient-related records (concurrently or retrospectively) to develop user (i.e., physician) profiles.

1.1.25 Confer with peers, providers, and/or users of departmental or institutional services.

1.1.26 Perform concurrent medical record review.

1.1.27 Participate in departmental and/or institutional committees.

1.1.28 Assign severity of illness categories.

1.1.30 Assign diagnostic/procedure codes using ICD-9-CM, CPT, HCPCS, DSM, or other coding systems.

Knowledge of:

K-1 Accreditation standards related to patient-related data (accreditation standards for various types of facilities)

K-2 Federal and state regulations related to patient-related data (regulations for various types of facilities)

K-5 Work measurement and analysis

K-6 Professional practice standards (i.e., AHIMA) and other related data (regulations for various types of facilities)

K-7 Quality control techniques

K-8 Disease process

K-9 Language of medicine (i.e., medical terminology)

K-10 Office ergonomics

K-11 Safety standards (i.e., OSHA, state, Joint Commission, etc.)

K-12 Legal requirements for confidentiality of patient-related data (federal and state)

K-13 Medical record content

K-14 Record/information control system

K-15 Vital statistics (i.e., state and federal regulations, and procedures for collection and reporting)

K-16 Communication techniques (oral: interpersonal, small group, professional speaking; written: business and professional writing)

K-17 Record filing systems

K-18 Healthcare facility organization

K-19 Healthcare facility committees (i.e., medical staff, administrative including Medical Record, Quality Assurance, Risk Management, etc.)

K-20 Business/committee procedures and rules of order

K-21 Case-mix systems (i.e., DRGs, APACHE, Medisgroups, etc.)

K-22 Medical nomenclatures and diagnostic classification systems (i.e., ICD-9-CM, CPT, HCPCS, DSM, etc.)

K-48 Cancer staging systems

Skill at:

S-1 Survey instrument design (i.e., written and interview)

S-2 Interviewing

S-5 Work measurement techniques

S-6 Quality control methods

S-7 Data presentation (manual and computer)

S-8 Data collection techniques

S-9 Data analysis

S-10 Interpretation of medical record content

S-11 Implementation of new/revised systems

S-12 Collection and compilation of vital statistics

S-13 Interpersonal and small group communications

S-14 Filing procedures (i.e., alphabetical, numerical)

S-17 Applying principles of diagnostic classification systems

S-18 Apply case-mix algorithms

S-19 Critical thinking

Tasks

1.2 Validate data for patient-related information systems needs, or for departmental operations or services.

Subtasks

1.2.1 Verify that data have been obtained from valid sources.

1.2.2 Verify timeliness, completeness, accuracy, and appropriateness of data sources (patient-care, management, billing reports, and/or databases).

1.2.3 Compare data with standards (i.e., length of stay norms, Medicare mortality rates, departmental productivity standards, etc.).

1.2.4 Check data for internal consistency.

1.2.5 Perform edit checks to monitor data accuracy.

1.2.6 Compare data with other data sources/references to determine consistency.

1.2.7 Validate diagnostic and procedure coding (i.e., ICD-9-CM, CPT, HCPCS, or other coding systems).

1.2.8 Validate DRG assignment.

Knowledge of:

K-1; K-2; K-7 - K-9; K-13 - K-15; K-19; K-21; K-22

K-23 Data verification techniques

K-24 Peer review organization standards/procedures

Skill at:

S-6; S-9; S-10; S-17; S-18

S-19 Critical thinking

Task

1.3 Analyze data for patient-related information system needs or for departmental operations or services.

Subtasks

1.3.1 Prepare data for analysis (i.e., compile data, develop graphs, tables, etc.).

1.3.2 Perform departmental/institutional case-mix analysis.

1.3.3 Analyze patient care data in relation to institutional performance standards.

1.3.4 Analyze patient care/institutional data in relation to regulatory and accreditation standards.

1.3.5 Analyze employee performance data in relation to departmental/institutional performance standards.

1.3.6 Analyze physician performance data/profiles in relation to medical staff, institutional, or regulatory, accreditation standards.

1.3.7 Analyze clinical or institutional data in relation to previous/current internal and external patterns to identify trends and patterns.

1.3.8 Calculate institutional statistics (i.e., occupancy rates, census, length of stay).

1.3.9 Apply statistical techniques for analyzing departmental/institutional/patient-related data (i.e., mean, standard deviation, variance, etc.).

1.3.10 Apply statistical techniques for determining data validity and reliability (i.e., chi square, Cronbach's alpha, etc.).

1.3.11 Analyze case-mix payment rates (i.e., DRG and others) to determine reimbursement optimization.

1.3.12 Analyze results of quality assurance, utilization review, risk management, and/or research studies.

Knowledge of:

K-1; K-2; K-5 - K-9; K-13; K-15; K-18 - K-22; K-24

K-25 Statistical techniques

K-26 Data presentation techniques

K-27 Research design

K-28 Computer statistical packages (i.e., SPSS, SAS, etc.)

K-29 Principles/methods for assessing patient-care quality and effectiveness

K-30 Principles/methods for assessing resources for patient care

K-31 Principles/methods of risk management

Skill at:

S-1; S-5; S-7 - S-10; S-18; S-19

S-20 Applying procedures for assessing patient-care quality/effectiveness

S-21 Interpretation of statistical data.

Domains, Tasks, and Subtasks

Domain 2

Design and select departmental service, operational, and information systems for patient-related data.

Task

2.1 Design departmental service and operational systems.

Subtasks

2.1.1 Develop departmental plans, goals, and objectives for areas under your span of control.

2.1.2 Determine feasibility and constraints applicable to design/redesign of departmental operational systems (i.e., costs, staffing, space, etc.)

2.1.3 Develop/revise departmental policies.

2.1.4 Develop/revise departmental procedures.

2.1.5 Develop/revise job descriptions.

2.1.6 Establish priorities for design/redesign of operational and/or information systems.

2.1.7 Pilot test new/revised systems.

2.1.8 Develop transition plans for implementation of new or revised systems.

2.1.9 Prepare budgets.

2.1.10 Design departmental operational systems for collection and processing of patient-related data (i.e., quantitative analysis, diagnostic and procedure coding, registries, etc.).

2.1.11 Design departmental operational systems for production control (i.e., establishing productivity levels, production monitoring, etc.).

2.1.12 Design departmental operational systems for information control (i.e., release of patient-related data, record tracking, etc.).

2.1.13 Design departmental operational systems for quality control (i.e., quality control of filing, coding, transcription, etc.).

2.1.14 Design departmental operational systems for information retention and retrieval (i.e., filing systems, filing equipment, retention policies/procedures, etc.).

2.1.15 Design ergonomically sound work environment.

2.1.16 Develop goals and objectives for computerized information systems (i.e., department or other facility systems).

2.1.17 Write functional specifications for computerized information systems (i.e., departmental or other facility systems).

2.1.18 Plan computerized system testing procedures (audit scripts) for computerized information systems (departmental or other systems).

2.1.19 Develop computerized system security procedures for computerized information systems (i.e., departmental or other systems).

2.1.20 Develop inservice education programs for departmental or non-departmental staff.

Knowledge of:

K-1 - K-7; K-10 - K-15; K-17 - K-19; K-21 - K-25; K-30; K-31

K-32 Management principles of planning and organizing

K-33 Functions related to Medical Record, Utilization Management, Quality Assurance, Cancer Registry, and related departments

K-34 Management principles of controlling

K-35 Business and professional writing techniques

K-36 Principles of job analysis

K-37 General systems principles

K-38 Work simplification techniques

K-39 Forms design and management

K-40 Information technologies

K-41 Systems analysis design, development, and implementation principles

K-42 Project planning

K-43 Data security techniques (Manual and Computer)

K-44 Space Management

K-45 Methods/procedures for procurement, maintenance, and selection of equipment and supplies

K-49 Principles of inservice education

Skill at:

S-3 - S-6; S-8; S-9; S-11; S-19 - S-21

S-22 Professional and business writing

S-23 Applying work simplification techniques

S-24 Systems analysis

S-25 Applying project planning techniques

S-26 Inservice education development and presentation

Domains, Tasks, and Subtasks

Task

2.2 Identify/select resources to support departmental operations and information systems.

Subtasks

2.2.1 Participate in preparation of requests for proposal bids for vendor services.

2.2.2 Evaluate vendor bids.

2.2.3 Review vendor contracts.

2.2.4 Negotiate contracts with vendors.

2.2.5 Prepare requests for proposal for vendor services.

2.2.6 Determine personnel needs for staffing current and/or new systems.

2.2.7 Determine equipment and/or supply needs for current and/or new systems.

2.2.8 Determine space requirements for current and/or new systems.

Knowledge of:

K-3; K-5; K-10; K-16 - K-17; K-33; K-36; K-39; K-40; K-44 - K-45

Skill at:

S-3; S-9; S-19; S-21; S-23

Domains, Tasks, and Subtasks

Domain 3

Implement departmental service and operational systems, and information systems for patient-related data.

Task

3.1 Execute plan(s) for implementing departmental service and operational systems, and information systems for patient-related data.

Subtasks

3.1.1 Select personnel.

3.1.2 Train personnel.

3.1.3 Inform organization staff of plan(s).

3.1.4 Implement new-revised policies and procedures.

3.1.5 Monitor adherence to system specifications.

3.1.6 Implement new/revised information, and/or service, and/or operational systems.

3.1.7 Monitor adherence to budget (i.e., determine budget variance, etc.).

3.1.8 Coordinate on-site review activities (i.e., PRO reviews, etc.).

3.1.9 Monitor policy/procedure compliance.

3.1.10 Counsel/discipline employees.

3.1.11 Terminate employees.

3.1.12 Design employee staffing schedules.

3.1.13 Maintain equipment (i.e., schedule preventive mainte-nance, arrange for repairs, etc.).

3.1.14 Educate medical record and/or other students assigned to the facility.

3.1.15 Conduct educational programs for departmental and/or non-departmental staff.

Knowledge of:

K-3 - K-5; K-16; K-18; K-32; K-33; K-34; K-35; K-45

K-46 Principles of human resources management

K-47 Principles of organizational behavior

K-49 Inservice education design and presentation

Skill at:

S-2; S-3; S-5; S-6; S-9; S-11; S-19; S-21; S-25; S-26

S-27 Applying principles of human resources manage-ment (i.e., selecting, training, motivating, promot-ing personnel, etc.)

Domains, Tasks, and Subtasks

Domain 4

Evaluate departmental, operational, and service systems, and information systems for patient-related data.

Task

4.1 Evaluate the effectiveness and efficiency of departmen-tal, operational and service systems, and information systems for patient-related data.

Subtasks

4.1.1 Monitor system outcomes (i.e., benefits, costs, etc.).

4.1.2 Determine variation(s) from established objectives and/or standards of performance.

4.1.3 Recommend changes and/or improvement(s) in sys-tems.

4.1.4 Evaluate employee performance.

Knowledge of:

K-1; K-2; K-6 - K-7; K-11 - K-17; K-19; K-21 - K-25; K-28 - K-40; K-43 - K-47

Skill at:

S-1 -S-2; S-5 - S-6; S-8; S-9; S-19; S-20 - S-22; S-27

KNOWLEDGE SKILLS AND CONTENT AREAS

This summary includes all certification examination knowledge and skill areas identified during the 1991 AHIMA Entry Level ART and RRA Job Analysis. While some of the Knowledge and Skill areas are the same for both entry level ARTs and RRAs, there are many differences for the two levels of practice. This document identifies the knowledge and skill areas. It does not imply that these areas are to be taught at the same level of complexity in both ART and RRA programs.

Knowledge Areas

K-1 Accreditation standards related to patient-related data (accreditation standards for various types of facilities)

K-2 Federal and state regulations related to patient-related data (regulations for various types of facilities)

K-3 Budgeting (i.e., budget types, procedures, principles)

K-4 Managerial accounting

K-5 Work measurement and analysis

K-6 Professional practice standards (i.e., AHIMA and others relating to patient-related data)

K-7 Quality control techniques

K-8 Disease process

K-9 Language of medicine (i.e., medical terminology)

K-10 Office ergonomics

K-11 Safety standards (i.e., OSHA, state, Joint Commission, etc.)

K-12 Legal requirements for confidentiality of patient-related data (federal and state)

K-13 Medical record content

K-14 Record/information control systems

K-15 Vital statistics (i.e., state and federal regulations, and procedures for collection and reporting)

K-16 Communication techniques (oral: interpersonal, small group, professional speaking; written: business and professional writing)

K-17 Record filing systems

K-18 Healthcare facility organization

K-19 Healthcare facility committees (i.e., medical staff, administrative including Medical Record, Quality Assurance, Risk Management, etc.)

K-20 Business/committee procedures and rules of order

K-21 Case-mix systems (i.e., DRGs, APACHE, Medisgroups, etc.)

K-22 Medical nomenclatures and diagnostic classification systems (i.e., ICD-9-CM, CPT, HCPCS, DSM, etc.)

K-23 Data verification techniques

K-24 Peer review organization standards/procedures

K-25 Statistical techniques

K-26 Data presentation techniques

K-27 Research design

K-28 Computer statistical packages (i.e., SPSS, SAS, etc.)

K-29 Principles/methods for assessing patient care quality and effectiveness

K-30 Principles/methods for assessing resources for patient care

K-31 Principles/methods of risk management

K-32 Management principles of planning and organizing

K-33 Functions related to Medical Record, Utilization Management, Quality Assurance, Cancer Registry, and related departments

K-34 Management principles of controlling

K-35 Business and professional writing techniques

K-36 Principles of job analysis

K-37 General systems principles

K-38 Work simplification techniques

K-39 Forms design and management

K-40 Information technologies

K-41 Systems analysis design, development and implementation principles

K-42 Project planning

K-43 Data security techniques (manual and computer)

K-44 Space management

K-45 Methods/procedures for procurement, maintenance, and selection of equipment and supplies

K-46 Principles of human resources management

K-47 Principles of organizational behavior

K-48 Cancer staging systems

K-49 Inservice education design and presentation

Skill Areas

S-1 Survey instrument design (i.e., written and interview)

S-2 Interviewing

S-3 Budget development and implementation

S-4 Application of managerial accounting techniques

S-5 Work measurement techniques

S-6 Quality control methods

S-7 Data presentation (manual and computer)

S-8 Data collection techniques

S-9 Data analysis

S-10 Interpretation of medical record content

S-11 Implementation of new/revised systems

S-12 Collection and compilation of vital statistics

S-13 Interpersonal and small group communications

S-14 Filing procedures (i.e., alphabetical, numerical)

S-15 Professional speaking and presentation

S-16 Conducting committee/business meetings

S-17 Applying principles of diagnostic classification systems

S-18 Apply case-mix algorithms

S-19 Critical thinking

S-20 Applying procedures for assessing patient care quality/effectiveness

S-21 Interpretation of statistical data

S-22 Professional and business writing

S-23 Applying work simplification techniques

S-24 Systems analysis

S-25 Applying project planning techniques

S-26 Inservice education development/presentation principles

S-27 Applying principles of human resources management (i.e., selecting, training, motivating, promoting personnel, etc.)

S-28 Cancer staging

Adopted by the Council on Certification

January 1992

Scheduled for implementation

Fall 1992

SECTION TWO

Review Questions by Chapter

HEALTH CARE SYSTEMS 1

PRETEST REVIEW

Directions:

1. Tear out a Pretest Review Answer Sheet from the back of this review manual.

2. Read each question carefully before selecting an answer.

3. Write the correct or best answer on the answer sheet.

4. Answer all the questions, since there is no penalty for this pretest review.

5. Check your answers with the answer key located near the end of this chapter.

1. The type of care provided to hospice patients is primarily curative care.

    a. True
    b. False

2. Both state and local governments are responsible for setting objectives for the attainment of goals explicated in the report: *Healthy People 2000*.

    a. True
    b. False

3. A completely electronic patient record will necessitate the electronic processing of information at the point of service.

    a. True
    b. False

4. The Medicare program is administered by the states.

    a. True
    b. False

5. The process of measuring a health care facility's compliance with established rules and regulations for Medicare and Medicaid reimbursement is called licensure.

    a. True
    b. False

6. The process of giving legal approval for a health care facility to operate is called certification. *volunta* *licensure involunta*

    a. True
    b. False

7. The authority to license health care facilities is vested in state government.

    a. True
    b. False

8. A copayment is a method of direct pay assumed by a subscriber in a managed care setting.

    a. True
    b. False

9. Medicaid reimbursement terms vary with each state.

   a. True
   b. False

10. Both the medical staff organization and the governing board of a hospital function according to respective bylaws.

    a. True
    b. False

11. The use of radioisotopes, such as a thyroid scan, is a diagnostic procedure conducted by diagnostic radiology services.

    a. True
    b. False

12. Hospice care reimbursement comes from Medicare and Medicaid only.

    a. True
    b. False

CHAPTER REVIEW

Directions:

1. Tear out a Chapter Review Answer Sheet from the back of this review manual.

2. Read each question carefully before selecting an answer.

3. Write the correct or best answer on the answer sheet.

4. Answer all the questions since there is no penalty in this chapter review.

5. Check your answers with the answer key located at the end of this chapter review.

1. Which of the following is *not* true about federal government regulation of health care?

    a. it investigates fraud and abuse arising from any health care facility or licensed physician
    b. it guarantees access to health care
    c. it enacts legislation impacting health care systems
    d. it owns and controls health care facilities

2. Which is *not* true about the organization structure of the DHHS?

    a. it includes the SSA
    b. it includes the Office of Inspector General
    c. it funds and coordinates regional offices
    d. it subsidizes the JCAHO

3. To be eligible for participation in the Medicare program and for financial reimbursement of its services, health care facilities must demonstrate compliance with the:

    a. *Conditions of Participation*
    b. *Essentials*
    c. standards of the JCAHO
    d. clinical practice guidelines

4. The certification of health care facilities for participation in the Medicare program is the responsibility of the states.

    a. True
    b. False

5. Which of the following is *not* true about state government regulation of health care?

    a. it operates public health departments
    b. it administers certification and licensing of health care practitioners
    c. it accredits home health and rehabilitation facilities
    d. it funds medical education through educational institutions

6. Physicians responsible for federally-funded patients in a certified health care facility are referred to as _____.

7. Every patient who arrives at a health care facility with an emergency medical condition must be evaluated to determine if the patient condition warrants therapy or transfer to another appropriate health care facility. This was mandated by which legislation?

    a. Occupational Safety and Health Act
    b. Consolidated Omnibus Budget Reconciliation Act
    c. Patient Self-Determination Act
    d. Omnibus Budget Reconciliation Act

8. A(n) _____ is a legal, written document that specifies patient preferences regarding future health care and especially in relation to resuscitation and life-extending measures.

9. Providers of care have been mandated to develop policies and procedures on the subject of self-determination.

    a. True
    b. False

10. _____ is the voluntary process by which an organization performs an external review and grants recognition to a program or health care facility that meets its predetermined standards.

11. Which is *not* an organization that sets voluntary standards for hospitals pertaining to quality health care?

    a. Department of Health and Human Services
    b. American Osteopathic Association
    c. Joint Commission on Accreditation of Health Care Organizations
    d. American College of Surgeons

12. "Deemed status" is a designation made by the JCAHO recognizing a health care facility's eligibility to receive Medicare funds.

    a. True
    b. False

13. Standards are published by the JCAHO for all of the following types of facilities *except:*

    a. planned parenthood organizations
    b. long term care organizations
    c. non-hospital psychiatric and substance abuse organizations
    d. ambulatory care organizations

14. The accrediting agency for rehabilitation facilities is:

    a. CARF
    b. CHAP
    c. AOA
    d. NLN

15. CAAHEP accredits allied health programs.

    a. True
    b. False

16. Services provided by health care facilities are generally directed to a geographic area called a point of service area.

    a. True
    b. False

17. What type of care is primarily provided to hospice patients?

    a. palliative
    b. curative
    c. diagnostic
    d. therapeutic

18. Point of service plans require patient subscribers to utilize a primary care physician as a gatekeeper.

    a. True
    b. False

19. Partnering is the ideal relationship between health care providers and contractors such as laundry, transcription, and physical therapy.

    a. True
    b. False

20. Physicians are licensed to practice by the:

    a. state
    b. Federation Licensing Examination
    c. National Board of Medical Examiners
    d. Accreditation Council on Graduate Medical Education

21. It is the responsibility of admitting services to assure that all health records document whether advanced directives have been signed by patients.

    a. True
    b. False

22. CAAHEP standards are called *Essentials* and are developed by the representative allied health organizations.

    a. True
    b. False

 # indirect pay involve the third party

23. *soft-pay* Out-of-pocket payment for health care is the same as direct pay.

    a. True
    b. False

24. A sliding scale payment method is commonly employed in managed health care settings.

    a. True
    b. False

25. When the cost of care is based on the patient's ability to pay it is referred to as a _sliding care fee_

26. Fee-for-service is a retrospective payment method.
    b pay based on provider's statement

    a. True
    b. False

27. Which is true of a prospective payment system?

    a. the amount of payment is fixed in advance of services
    b. the amount is based on the providers statement of cost *fee for ser, retrospective*
    c. it is the designated payment method for all inpatients and outpatients
    d. it is the designated payment according to the patient's ability to pay

28. A _fiscal_ is that organization which has contracted with the federal government to process Medicare claims and payments.

29. Native Americans and retired military personnel (including their dependents) are provided health care through CHAMPUS.

    a. True
    b. False

30. A _gate keeper_ is a primary care physician who participates in a managed care plan and is chiefly responsible for most of the care provided the enrollee.

31. When patient average length of stay is greater than *30* 20 days, the facility is classified by the AHA as a long term care facility.

    a. True
    b. False

32. A reimbursement method that is a prepaid, fixed amount to a provider per person served is:

    a. direct pay
    b. copayment
    c. capitation
    d. fee-for-service

33. Large hospitals in which health information systems embrace the financial, administrative and clinical information needs of the facility, health information management most likely would report to which officer?

    a. CEO
    b. CFO
    c. CIO *chief info officer*
    d. COO

34. The organizational structure of the medical staff in a 250 bed hospital would most likely include which of the following:

    a. officers
    b. committees
    c. clinical services
    d. all of the above

35. The professional staff organization of a hospital refers to the medical and other credentialed staff where permitted by state law.

    a. True
    b. False

Match each term in the left column with the correct descriptors in the right column. Not all descriptors may have answers.

d or __e__   36. acute care

__b__   37. ambulatory care   *, d*

____   38. inpatient care

____   39. (hospice care)

____   40. long term care ✓

____   41. managed care

____   42. outpatient care

____   43. palliative care

____   44. primary care

__g__   45. secondary care

____   46. tertiary care

a. general, coordinated care (except that requiring a specialist occurring in an ambulatory setting)

b. a patient receiving health services at a hospital without being hospitalized

c. highly specialized care provided by specialists

d. care rendered by an HMO, IPO or PPO

e. short term care to inpatients or outpatients

f. patient receiving health care services while provided room, board and continuous nursing service

g. health care services provided by a specialist at the request of the primary care physician

h. health care provided in a convalescent inpatient setting

i. process of assessing and sorting patients to determine priority for care

j. health care services that relieve symptoms or discomforts but are not curative

k. palliative and supportive care of the terminally ill

l. health care provided in an outpatient setting

m. care of a diagnostic and/or therapeutic nature provided to inpatients and outpatients

47. A health care system composed of two or more hospitals that are owned, managed or leased by a single organization are called a _____ .

48. Physical rehabilitation services includes each of the following *except:*

    a. occupational therapy
    b. speech therapy
    c. respiratory therapy
    d. physical therapy

PRETEST REVIEW ANSWER KEY

Directions:

1. Correct your Pretest Review—Answer Sheet with the answers below by placing a slash (Example: 8) through the incorrect question number with a pen or pencil of a contrasting color.

2. Record the correct answer to the right of your answer on your answer sheet.

3. Record the total correct on the Initial Performance Grid in section four of this review manual.

4. Calculate your performance rate and also record on the grid.

5. Promptly locate the correct answer for each question missed in the chapter of the textbook.

6. Proceed to the chapter review if your performance rate was 80% or higher, otherwise, return to the chapter for further study.

1.	b	5.	b	9.	a
2.	a	6.	b	10.	a
3.	a	7.	a	11.	b
4.	b	8.	a	12.	b

CHAPTER REVIEW ANSWER KEY

Directions:

1. Correct your Chapter Review-Answer Sheet with the answers below by placing a slash (Example: 8) through the incorrect question number with a pen or pencil of a contrasting color.

2. Record the correct answer to the right of your answer on your answer sheet.

3. Record the total correct on the Initial Performance Grid in section four of this review manual.

4. Calculate your performance rate and also record on the grid.

5. Promptly locate the correct answer for each question missed in the chapter of the textbook.

6. Proceed to the next assigned chapter in your study.

1.	b	6.	participating physicians	11.	a
2.	d	7.	b	12.	b
3.	a	8.	advance directive or living will	13.	a
4.	a	9.	a	14.	a
5.	c	10.	Accreditation	15.	b

16.	b	27.	a	38.	f
17.	a	28.	fiscal intermediary	39.	k
18.	a	29.	b	40.	h
19.	a	30.	gatekeeper	41.	d
20.	a	31.	b	42.	b or l
21.	b	32.	c	43.	j
22.	a	33.	c	44.	a or l
23.	a	34.	d	45.	g
24.	b	35.	a	46.	c or m
25.	sliding scale fee	36.	d or e	47.	multihospital system
26.	a	37.	b, d or ;	48.	c

THE HEALTH INFORMA-
TION MANAGEMENT
PROFESSION 2

PRETEST REVIEW

Directions:

1. Tear out a Pretest Review Answer Sheet from the back of this review manual.

2. Read each question carefully before selecting an answer.

3. Write the correct or best answer on the answer sheet.

4. Answer all the questions, since there is no penalty for this pretest review.

5. Check your answers with the answer key located near the end of this chapter..

1. The first minimum standards pertaining to the delivery of health care were established by the American Hospital Association. USHHS

   a. True
   b. False

2. Early hospital accreditation activities were shared by several organizations including the American Dental Association.

   a. True
   b. False

3. The format of the patient record was significantly changed by the Tax Equity and Fiscal Responsibility Act.

   a. True
   b. False

4. The health record is the source document to verify the reimbursement of care.

   a. True
   b. False

5. The Computer-Based Record Institute is a non-member organization.

   a. True
   b. False

6. AHIMA plays an active role in the development of standards by other organizations.

   a. True
   b. False

7. JCAHO and AHIMA standards are revised annually.

   a. True
   b. False

8. The health record is influenced by standards and regulations arising from non-governmental and governmental agencies.

   a. True
   b. False

9. Early educational programs in medical records were largely located in hospitals.

    a. True
    b. False

10. There have been two levels of formal education programs since the inception of the professional association — medical record technology and medical record administration.

    a. True
    b. False

11. Since 1944 there have been two medical record associations in North America.

    a. True
    b. False

12. Recertification is a requirement for all credentialed practitioners in the medical/health record profession.

    a. True
    b. False

CHAPTER REVIEW

Directions:

1. Tear out a Chapter Review —Answer Sheet from the back of this review manual.

2. Read each question carefully before selecting an answer.

3. Write the correct or best answer on the answer sheet.

4. Answer all the questions since there is no penalty in this chapter review.

5. Check your answers with the answer key located at the end of this chapter review.

1. When did the recording of clinical information begin in the U.S.?

    a. late 1700's
    b. early 1800's
    c. late 1800's
    d. early 1900's

2. The earliest medical records in the U.S. were:

    a. letter formatted
    b. ledger formatted
    c. formatted by patient
    d. catalogued by diseases and operations

3. The initial organization of practitioners in medical records referred to themselves as 'librarians' because they viewed themselves as custodians of the medical record.

    a. True
    b. False

4. The findings of the Flexner Report promoted the primary patient record as a source for quality care assessment.

    a. True
    b. False

5. Which organization actively demonstrated the need for quality patient records in the early 1900's?

    a. ACS
    b. AHA
    c. AMRA
    d. JCAH

6. One condition of participation in the Medicare/Medicaid program is the willingness of health care providers to submit to comprehensive review activities.

    a. True
    b. False

7. Early standards in health care specified certain documentation within a stated time and certain content of the patient record.

    a. True
    b. False

8. The accreditation process for hospitals in the early part of the century was involuntary and pertained to surgery.

    a. True
    b. False

9. The use of DRGs for reimbursement of care was implemented in l965.

    a. True
    b. False

10. The assignment of the DRG for Medicare reimbursement is determined after patient discharge.

    a. True
    b. False

11. The DRG reimbursement system applies to all Medicare and non-Medicare patients in all states. *medicare only*

    a. True
    b. False

12. Hospitals complying with JCAHO standards are automatically deemed compliant with state licensing regulations in all 50 states. *every state are different*

    a. True
    b. False

13. Hospitals complying with JCAHO standards are automatically deemed compliant with the *Conditions of Participation*.

    a. True
    b. False

14. Licensing health care institutions is a function of state government.

    a. True
    b. False

15. Fee-for-service reimbursement has been replaced by fixed rate reimbursement for all Medicare and Medicaid patients.

    a. True
    b. False

16. The first educational program for medical record librarians was founded in 1929. *1954*

    a. True
    b. False

17. Which standards apply to the approval process of medical record/health information education programs?

    a. essentials *& the' thisis*
    b. regulations
    c. *Conditions of Participation*
    d. none of the above

18. The correspondence program, now called the Independent Study Program, was made available as an alternative to the school-based programs in both medical record technology and medical record administration.

    a. True
    b. False

19. Between 1943 and 1994 the accreditation of educational programs in medical records was a cooperative effort with the American Hospital Association.

    a. True
    b. False

20. Utilization of services and the quality of care rendered to Medicare patients are monitored by internal review constituencies on behalf of HCFA.

    a. True
    b. False

21. Incentives for health care reimbursement were altered by the IOM Report in 1991.

    a. True
    b. False

22. The actual cost of care rendered to patients is the same as the DRG rate and can be determined before admission for most Medicare patients.

    a. True
    b. False

23. The DRG reimbursement is based on the patient's length of stay and utilization of services.

    a. True
    b. False

24. The clinical record is the principal source of reimbursement information.

    a. True
    b. False

clingers' chick

25. Capitated care was a step towards changing the incentives in health care.

    a. True
    b. False

26. The formal organization of medical record workers transpired in ___1928___.

27. What was the name given to the initial organization currently named AHIMA?

    a. Association of Record Librarians of North America
    b. American Association of Record Librarians
    c. Association of Medical Record Clerks
    d. American Association of Medical Record Workers

28. By 1939, a majority of the states had state or local organizations which were affiliated with the national association of medical record practitioners.

    a. True
    b. False

29. The official publication of the initial organization of medical record workers was published bi-monthly.

    a. True
    b. False

30. Certification of education program graduates by examination commenced in 1933.

    a. True
    b. False

31. After l959, registration of a medical record librarian was not based on work experience and formal education.

    a. True
    b. False

32. Registration replaced the process of certifying program graduates in 1959.

    a. True
    b. False

33. The credential — CRL — was to registered medical record librarians as "fellow" is to a physician, presently.

    a. True
    b. False

34. Which of the following credentials is presently awarded by AHIMA?

    a. ART
    b. CCS
    c. RRA
    d. all of the above

35. The reimbursement payment method for care rendered to Medicare and Medicaid inpatients is fee-for-service in most states.

    a. True
    b. False

36. At its inception, the JCAH was comprised of which of the following:

    a. ACS
    b. AHA
    c. The Canadian Hospital Association
    d. all of the above

37. Early accreditation activities focused on private physician practices and charitable hospitals.

    a. True
    b. False

38. In the l920's, the patient record was a source of needed information for board certification by the American College of Surgeons.

    a. True
    b. False

39. Compliance with state licensing requirements is mandatory in all states.

    a. True
    b. False

40. AHIMA sets standards for health records in addition to JCAHO standards.

    a. True
    b. False

41. Facilities have the freedom to develop what they need as a health record using regulations and standards to guide the process and outcome.

    a. True
    b. False

42. Institutional providers of care may voluntarily opt for compliance with regulations pertaining to Medicare and Medicaid.

    a. True
    b. False

43. Compliance with JCAHO standards is voluntary for health care organizations.

    a. True
    b. False

44. Prior to the association's name being changed to AHIMA, it was recognized as the ___AMRA___.

45. The organization structure of AHIMA is comprised of 50 component state associations plus associations in the District of Columbia, Puerto Rico and Mexico.

    a. True
    b. False

46. Which is *not* a volunteer policy-setting structure of AHIMA?

    a. executive director
    b. board of directors
    c. house of delegates
    d. councils
    e. none of the above

47. AHIMA members elect each of the following except the:

    a. executive director
    b. board of directors
    c. council on certification
    d. nominating committee

48. In the practice of health information management, health information professionals are bound by a code of ethics which expressly prohibits illegal, incompetent and unethical acts.

    a. True
    b. False

PRETEST REVIEW ANSWER KEY

Directions:

1. Correct your Pretest Review Answer Sheet with the answers below by placing a slash (Example: ✗) through the incorrect question number with a pen or pencil of a contrasting color.

2. Record the correct answer to the right of your answer on your answer sheet.

3. Record the total correct on the Initial Performance Grid in section four of this review manual.

4. Calculate your performance rate and also record on the grid.

5. Promptly locate the correct answer for each question missed in the chapter of the textbook.

6. Proceed to the chapter review if your performance rate was 80% or higher, otherwise, return to the chapter for further study.

1.	b	5.	b	9.	a
2.	a	6.	a	10.	b
3.	b	7.	b	11.	a
4.	a	8.	a	12.	b

CHAPTER REVIEW ANSWER KEY

Directions:

1. Correct your Chapter Review-Answer Sheet with the answers below by placing a slash (Example: ✗) through the incorrect question number with a pen or pencil of a contrasting color.

2. Record the correct answer to the right of your answer on your answer sheet.

3. Record the total correct on the Initial Performance Grid in section four of this review manual.

4. Calculate your performance rate and also record on the grid.

5. Promptly locate the correct answer for each question missed in the chapter of the textbook.

6. Proceed to the next assigned chapter in your study.

1.	b	6.	a	11.	b
2.	b	7.	a	12.	b
3.	a	8.	b	13.	a
4.	b	9.	b	14.	a
5.	a	10.	a	15.	b

16.	b	27.	a	39.	a
17.	a	28.	a	40.	a
18.	b	29.	b	41.	a
19.	b	30.	b	42.	a
20.	b	31.	a	43.	a
21.	b	32.	b	44.	American Medical Record Association (AMRA)
22.	b	33.	a		
23.	b	34.	d	45.	b
24.	a	35.	b	46.	a
25.	a	36.	d	47.	a
26.	1928	37.	b	48.	a
		38.	a		

PATIENT AND HEALTH CARE DATA

3

PRETEST REVIEW

Directions:

1. Tear out a Pretest Review Answer Sheet from the back of this review manual.

2. Read each question carefully before selecting an answer.

3. Write the correct or best answer on the answer sheet.

4. Answer all the questions, since there is no penalty for this pretest review.

5. Check your answers with the answer key located near the end of this chapter

1. Standards formulated by agencies called practice guidelines are not enforceable.

    a. True
    b. False

2. Timeliness in data collection refers to capturing the data at the moment patient care is rendered.

    a. True
    b. False

3. Diagnostic and procedure indexes are a source of primary data.

    Secondary

    a. True
    b. False

4. The UHDDS was first developed by the JCAHO.

    a. True
    b. False

5. Data sets standardize both the data collected and the information reported for comparative purposes.

    a. True
    b. False

6. The Omnibus Reconciliation Act of 1987 mandated the use of the Minimum Data Set for long term care.

    a. True
    b. False

7. A patient information system should include data controls for detecting the location of errors in addition to detecting errors in validity.

    a. True
    b. False

8. PROs are required to evaluate the quality of care provided to hospital inpatients and outpatients.

    a. True
    b. False

9. Utilization review personnel collect data relative to a facility's efficiency.

   a. True
   b. False

10. Current JCAHO standards require hospitals to use computer technology in the collection of information.

    a. True
    b. False

11. Hospital census data are types of vital statistics.

    a. True
    b. False

12. Morbidity refers to cause of death data.

    a. True
    b. False

CHAPTER REVIEW

Directions:

1. Tear out a Chapter Review Answer Sheet from the back of this review manual.

2. Read each question carefully before selecting an answer.

3. Write the correct or best answer on the answer sheet.

4. Answer all the questions since there is no penalty in this chapter review.

5. Check your answers with the answer key located at the end of this chapter review.

1. The UHDDS is a data set used for abstracting hospital-based outpatient care.

   a. True
   b. False

2. A fiscal intermediary processes Medicare reimbursement claims.

   a. True
   b. False

3. The extent to which data meet the goals and needs of an organization refers to its appropriateness.

   a. True
   b. False

4. Which is not a data element included in the MDS?

   a. cognition
   b. daily patterns of activity
   c. principal procedure
   d. psychosocial status

5. The judicial process uses _____ to settle an injury case involving an automobile accident.

   a. aggregate data
   b. primary data
   c. case mix data
   d. registry data

6. Blue Cross/Blue Shield uses _____ to resolve a claim for payment.

   a. primary data
   b. case mix data
   c. both a and b
   d. neither a nor b

7. Patients use _____ to research their genetic history.

   a. primary data
   b. case mix data
   c. registry data
   d. secondary data

8. The media uses _____ to report on health information of epidemiologic interest to the public such as a tuberculosis outbreak.

   a. primary data
   b. clinical data
   c. aggregate data
   d. none of the above

9. Which organization does not promulgate standards or regulations relating to data quality management?

   a. AHIMA
   b. HCFA
   c. PPO
   d. JCAHO

10. Providers use health care information for

    a. reimbursement of services
    b. evaluation of care
    c. education of staff
    d. all of the above

11. The storage and retrieval of information from a database is accomplished by a database management system.

    a. True
    b. False

12. Which is a software program for tracking the utilization of services in managed care settings?

    a. Ambulatory Care Group Case Mix Management System
    b. Clinical Information Management System
    c. Uniform Clinical Data Set
    d. Uniform Ambulatory Care Data Set

Match the terms in the left column with the correct discriptor in the right column. Not all descriptors may have answers.

_k_ 13. data

_i_ 14. information

_e_ 15. primary data

_h or b_ 16. secondary data

_g_ 17. accurate data

_f_ 18. cost effective data

_b or h_ 19. aggregate data

_j_ 20. reimbursement data

_c_ 21. clinical data

_d_ 22. confidential data

a. data elements that describe patient characteristics such as DOB, race, sex

b. grouped data or data elements regarding several individuals

c. data related to medical/surgical care

d. identified/privileged data

e. data originating at the source of care

f. the value of data exceeds the cost of its collection and dissemination

g. valid data

h. data in an index or register are an example

i. processed facts and figures

j. data including financial guarantor for services

k. raw facts and figures

l. data about a particular aspect of health care delivery such as trauma, implants, and organ sharing organized into a database

23. The term "demographics" is often used in reference to what type of data?

    a. financial
    b. socioeconomic
    c. clinical
    d. primary

24. A variety of departments in hospitals must use the same healthcare data. This requires that patient information systems:

    a. be purchased from the same vendor
    b. be developed by the same computer systems designer
    c. must be interfaced or integrated
    d. contain only primary data

25. Which of the following collects discharge data on federally-funded patients?

    a. Minimum Data Set
    b. National Practitioner Data Bank
    c. Resident Assessment Protocol
    d. Uniform Hospital Discharge Data Set

26. Which data set was developed for capturing primary data on outpatients and clinic patients for example?

    a. Uniform Clinical Data Set
    b. Uniform Ambulatory Care Data Set
    c. Ambulatory Care Group Case Mix Management System
    d. Minimum Data Set

27. One of the primary goals of the United Network of Organ Sharing is:

    a. to ensure organs are available for persons who are in need
    b. to provide for the distribution of organs
    c. to provide governmental control of organs
    d. to inform providers of available organs

28. Health care data of particular interest to the administration include:

    a. physicians orders
    b. patient address
    c. consultations
    d. services used

29. The organization that compiles data on osteopathic physician location and type of practice is the:

    a. JCAHO
    b. NPDB
    c. APA
    d. AOA

30. PSROs were replaced by PROs by the Tax Equity and Fiscal Responsibility Act of 1982.

    a. AOA
    b. AMA
    c. AHA
    d. JCAHO

31. Which is an organization that provides a comprehensive package of health care services for a fixed rate?

    a. health maintenance organization
    b. peer review organization
    c. preferred provider organization
    d. both a and c

32. The WEDI report focused on:

    a. reduction of costs through electronic claims processing
    b. educational programs regarding electronic data interchange
    c. standards for data content and coding structures
    d. vendor interfacing

33. The Resident Assessment Protocol is part of the Minimum Data Set for use in long term care.

    a. True
    b. False

34. The NAHDO was established to promote the availability of quality data for health care policy and research.

    a. True
    b. False

35. All clinical data is considered confidential according to AHIMA standards.

    a. True
    b. False

36. Which registry collects data internationally?

    a. cancer
    b.) implant
    c. organ sharing
    d. trauma

37. There is a national cancer database designed to collect data on the incidence, mortalit,y and survival of patients with cancer.

    a.) True
    b. False

38. The AMA has developed standards for emergency care and hospital cancer programs.

    a. True
    b.) False

39. The abbreviation ANSI represents the _American National Standards Institute_

40. PPOs direct a volume of patients to a specific provider for a reduced fee to its subscribers.

    a.) True
    b. False

41. The abbreviation, _EDI_, refers to the ability to exchange data electronically.

42. A computer validity check can identify unreasonable values in a given circumstance such as an unreasonably high laboratory value that would have a zero chance of ever occurring.

    a. True
    b.) False

43. The _____ developed the UHDDS.

44. The _ACS_ sets standards for the collection of cancer data by hospitals.

45. The purpose of the _HL7_ organization is to provide guidelines for interfacing health information systems within health care organizations or facilities.

46. Requiring the use of passwords to access a computerized data system is mandated for data protection.

    a. True
    b. False

47. Standards pertaining to the CPR are developed by which organization?

    a.) ASTM
    b. DHHS
    c. JCAHO
    d. HCFA

48. Which of the following is not associated with creating standards for the electronic exchange of healthcare data?

    a. HL7
    b. X12N
    c. ASTM
    d.) NPDB

PRETEST REVIEW ANSWER KEY

Directions:

1. Correct your Pretest Review—Answer Sheet with the answers below by placing a slash (Example:⁄8) through the incorrect question number with a pen or pencil of a contrasting color.

2. Record the correct answer to the right of your answer on your answer sheet.

3. Record the total correct on the Initial Performance Grid in section four of this review manual.

4. Calculate your performance rate and also record on the grid.

5. Promptly locate the correct answer for each question missed in the chapter of the textbook.

6. Proceed to the chapter review if your performance rate was 80% or higher, otherwise, return to the chapter for further study.

1.	a	5.	a	9.	a
2.	b	6.	a	10.	b
3.	b	7.	a	11.	b
4.	b	8.	b	12.	b

CHAPTER REVIEW ANSWER KEY

Directions:

1. Correct your Chapter Review-Answer Sheet with the answers below by placing a slash (Example:⁄8) through the incorrect question number with a pen or pencil of a contrasting color.

2. Record the correct answer to the right of your answer on your answer sheet.

3. Record the total correct on the Initial Performance Grid in section four of this review manual.

4. Calculate your performance rate and also record on the grid.

5. Promptly locate the correct answer for each question missed in the chapter of the textbook.

6. Proceed to the next assigned chapter in your study.

1.	b	6.	c	11.	a
2.	a	7.	a	12.	a
3.	a	8.	c	13.	k
4.	c	9.	c	14.	i
5.	b	10.	d	15.	e

16.	h or b	28.	d	40.	a
17.	g	29.	d	41.	EDI
18.	f	30.	b	42.	b
19.	b or h	31.	d	43.	U.S. Dept. of Health, Education & Welfare *now* U.S. Dept. of Health & Human Services or NCVHS
20.	j	32.	a		
21.	c	33.	b		
22.	d	34.	a		
23.	b	35.	a	44.	American College of Surgeons (ACS)
24.	c	36.	b		
25.	d	37.	a	45.	HL7
26.	b	38.	b	46.	b
27.	b	39.	American National Standards Institute	47.	a
				48.	d

DATA COLLECTION **4**

PRETEST REVIEW

Directions:

1. Tear out a Pretest Review Answer Sheet from the back of this review manual.

2. Read each question carefully before selecting an answer.

3. Write the correct or best answer on the answer sheet.

4. Answer all the questions, since there is no penalty for this pretest review.

5. Check your answers with the answer key located near the end of this chapter.

1. The smallest unit of data that can be stored in a computer system is called a data item.

    a. True
    b. False

2. Data can be processed electronically in the form of characters and numbers only.

    a. True
    b. False

3. When validating input, performance tests, and checks ensure that the input operation was legal and the input itself was reasonable.

    a. True
    b. False

4. Systems are interfaced when the functioning of one ends and another begins at a shared boundary between the systems.

    a. True
    b. False

5. Data have reliability when they are meaningful and relevant to their stated purpose.

    a. True
    b. False

6. All scanners are data input devices.

    a. True
    b. False

7. Standardized data sets such as the UHDDS employ data items accompanied by uniform definitions.

    a. True
    b. False

8. Data should be collected for a pre-specified, identified purpose irrespective of possible users.

    a. True
    b. False

9. In a CPR, the processing cycle begins with electronic input.

   a. True
   b. False

10. Graphical user interfaces control data output.

   a. True
   b. False

11. Audit trails ensure the processing of all items by adding numbers in a specific data field.

   a. True
   b. False

12. Invalid data can be traced back to their origin for correction by employing a transaction validation.

   a. True
   b. False

CHAPTER REVIEW

Directions:

1. Tear out a Chapter Review Answer Sheet from the back of this review manual.

2. Read each question carefully before selecting an answer.

3. Write the correct or best answer on the answer sheet.

4. Answer all the questions since there is no penalty in this chapter review.

5. Check your answers with the answer key located at the end of this chapter review.

1. Which is *not* a data set?

    a. UMLS
    b. LTCDS
    c. UACDS
    d. UHDDS

2. The purpose of encryption is the protection of sensitive data items such as the UPIN.

    a. True
    b. False

3. In a CPR, each data item should have a specified, authorized user(s).

    a. True
    b. False

4. A terminal is an example of a keyed data entry device.

    a. True
    b. False

5. Data entry devices must be compatible with the formatted data item.

    a. True
    b. False

6. Data validation in the CPR can precede or follow data entry.

    a. True
    b. False

7. Event validation in a CPR focuses on the acceptability of the transaction processing such as entering a record.

    a. True
    b. False

8. Event validation techniques include:

    a. audit trails
    b. batch totaling
    c. transaction validation
    d. all of the above

9. Which is *not* a relevant consideration when deciding the format of a form or computer screen view?

    a. regulations and standards regarding the record and needed content
    b. record linkage
    c. technology
    d. users

10. The Unified Medical Language System is a source of standardized data items and vocabularies.

   a. True
   b. False *(circled)*

11. Re-entering data is the duplicate processing of data for the purpose of input validation.

   a. True *(circled)*
   b. False

12. Which is *not* a format check?

   a. values *(circled)*
   b. processing codes
   c. type specification
   d. data length

13. Which is *not* included in the electronic validation of data?

   a. format checks
   b. check digits
   c. reasonableness checks
   d. sequence checks *(circled)*

14. Computer logs are a product of:

   a. duplicate processing
   b. audit trail validation *(circled)*
   c. batch totaling
   d. hash totaling

15. The "hash total" method of input validation examines fields of numbers.

   a. True
   b. False *(circled)*

16. UHDDS, ASTM E 1384, and MDS are mandatory data sets in health information systems.

   a. True
   b. False *(circled)*

17. The process of ensuring that a processing event is acceptable, authorized, and legitimate is called

   ~~transaction~~ validation *(handwritten)*

18. Referring to the form on the facing page, specify the footer information.

   approved OMB No. 0938 *(handwritten)*

19. Referring to the form on the facing page, is the footer located in the proper position according to accepted paper forms design principles?

   a. Yes
   b. No *(circled)*

20. Referring to the form on the facing page, is header information identifiable?

   a. Yes
   b. No *(circled)*

21. Referring to the form on the facing page, what segment of information is missing that is foundational to paper forms design?

   instruction or header *(handwritten)*

22. Edition dates on paper forms are part of the closing segment.

   a. True
   b. False *(circled)*

23. When a laboratory value falls outside a specified range, its outlier detection is a result of a:

   a. check digit
   b. format check
   c. reasonableness check *(circled)*
   d. sequence check

24. Computer view designs include menus.

   a. True *(circled)*
   b. False

25. Paper forms should include:

   a. instructions *(circled)*
   b. purpose
   c. user(s)
   d. controls

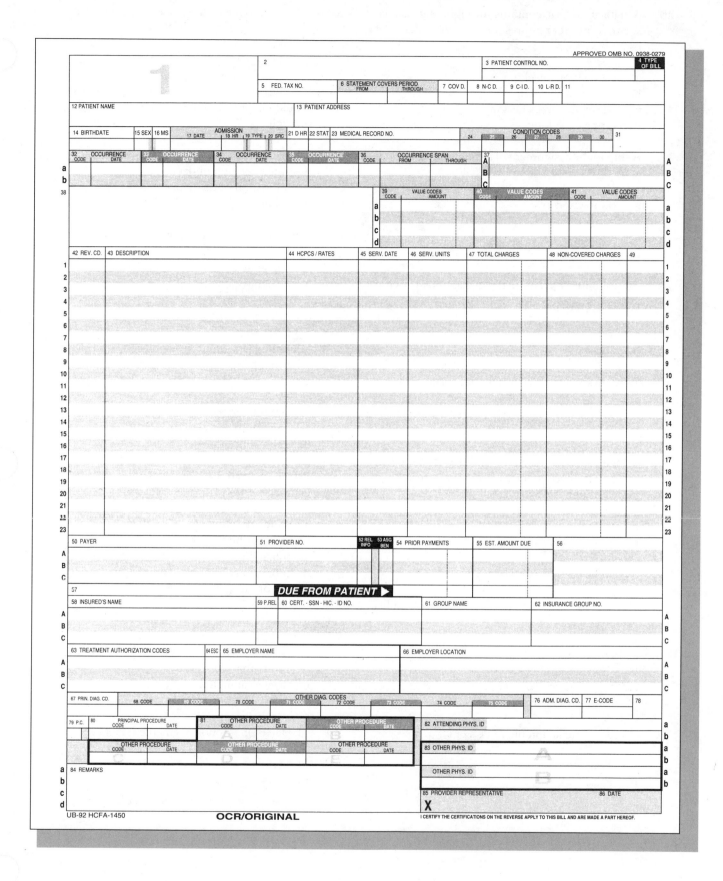

26. A data item that contains an eight-digit social security number represents an error detected by:

   a. transaction checking
   b. sequence checking
   c. reasonableness checking
   d. format checking

27. A skip in the assignment of admission numbers is a:

   a. transaction error
   b. batch error
   c. sequence error
   d. digit error

28. Computer views require the development of controls such as overrides.

   a. True
   b. False

29. Windows is a computer interface format.

   a. True
   b. False

30. Which validation check would detect at the moment of database contact an unauthorized attempt to delete a physician order?

   a. transaction
   b. reasonableness
   c. format
   d. audit trail

31. Transposition of a patient medical record number can be detected by a:

   a. check digit
   b. sequencing check
   c. format check
   d. transaction check

32. Windows are adaptable to PCs only.

   a. True
   b. False

33. Icons and tool bars are associated with GUIs.

   a. True
   b. False

34. Well-designed paper forms and computer views should guide the data collection process of users through:

   a. data entry
   b. interpretation of data
   c. validation of the data entered
   d. all of the above

35. Which is *not* a general format of the PPR?

   a. integrated
   b. patient-oriented
   c. problem-oriented
   d. source-oriented

36. Minimum data sets are available for use in all of the following health care delivery systems *except*:

   a. acute care
   b. ambulatory care
   c. long term care
   d. mental health care

37. Which characteristic qualifies the purposes of a data set?

   a. comparability
   b. compatibility
   c. reliability
   d. uniformity
   e. all of the above

38. The UPIN is used for:

   a. sequencing data
   b. formatting data
   c. event validation
   d. identification

39. The UHDDS is a non-segmented data set.

   a. True
   b. False

40. The U.S. Census Bureau plays an active role in sponsoring, developing and approving data sets in health care.

    a. True
    b. False

41. A _bottle neck_ _____occurs when certain operations in processing data begin to lag behind.

42. An integrated PPR is formatted by:

    a. date
    b. source
    c. problem
    d. none of the above

43. Health information management control issues in data collection should include:

    a. controlling costs
    b. identifying all views and forms
    c. capturing all the data
    d. all of the above

44. Shading a section of data in paper forms design is preferred over bordering and screening.

    a. True
    b. False

45. Rules structure a form by dividing in into logical sections.

    a. True
    b. False

46. Locating errors in the content of data items or fields is:

    a. data validation
    b. entry validation
    c. forms control
    d. reasonableness check

47. The ability to electronically link related records regarding a single patient is called:

    a. data interchange
    b. record linkage
    c. system integration
    d. system interfacing

48. Maintaining the confidentiality of the data is a management control issue.

    a. True
    b. False

PRETEST REVIEW ANSWER KEY

Directions:

1. Correct your Pretest Review Answer Sheet with the answers below by placing a slash (Example: 8) through the incorrect question number with a pen or pencil of a contrasting color.

2. Record the correct answer to the right of your answer on your answer sheet.

3. Record the total correct on the Initial Performance Grid in section four of this review manual.

4. Calculate your performance rate and also record on the grid.

5. Promptly locate the correct answer for each question missed in the chapter of the textbook.

6. Proceed to the chapter review if your performance rate was 80% or higher, otherwise, return to the chapter for further study.

1.	a	5.	b	9.	a
2.	b	6.	a	10.	b
3.	b	7.	a	11.	b
4.	a	8.	b	12.	b

CHAPTER REVIEW ANSWER KEY

Directions:

1. Correct your Chapter Review Answer Sheet with the answers below by placing a slash (Example: 8) through the incorrect question number with a pen or pencil of a contrasting color.

2. Record the correct answer to the right of your answer on your answer sheet.

3. Record the total correct on the Initial Performance Grid in section four of this review manual.

4. Calculate your performance rate and also record on the grid.

5. Promptly locate the correct answer for each question missed in the chapter of the textbook.

6. Proceed to the next assigned chapter in your study.

1.	a	6.	b	11.	a
2.	a	7.	a	12.	a
3.	a	8.	d	13.	d
4.	a	9.	b	14.	b
5.	b	10.	b	15.	b

16.	b	27.	c	38.	d
17.	transaction validation	28.	a	39.	a
18.	approved OMB No. 0938	29.	a	40.	b
19.	b	30.	a	41.	bottleneck
20.	b	31.	a	42.	a
21.	instructions and/or header	32.	b	43.	d
22.	b	33.	a	44.	b
23.	c	34.	d	45.	a
24.	a	35.	b	46.	a
25.	a	36.	d	47.	b
26.	d	37.	e	48.	a

DATA QUALITY 5

PRETEST REVIEW

Directions:

1. Tear out a Pretest Review Answer Sheet from the back of this review manual.

2. Read each question carefully before selecting an answer.

3. Write the correct or best answer on the answer sheet.

4. Answer all the questions, since there is no penalty for this pretest review.

5. Check your answers with the answer key located near the end of this chapter.

1. Testing the "restore" capabilities of a system is a mechanism for verifying backup system ability.

   a. True
   b. False

2. Categorical data in a database includes ICD-9-CM codes.

   a. True
   b. False

3. Date, time, and logic are types of fields in a database.

   a. True
   b. False

4. When an error in a computerized record is corrected, the system should preserve the corrected entry, not the original entry.

   a. true
   b. false

5. Narrative information can be a type of data field used in a database.

   a. True
   b. false

6. In a database, a column is a data field.

   a. true
   b. false

7. All the data about a single patient in a computer database system are called a file.

   a. true
   b. false

8. Point of service documentation issues pertain to computerized patient records and not to paper patient records.

   a. true
   b. false

9. Verifying the date of authentication is extremely difficult or impossible in paper records.

   a. true
   b. false

10. When setting up computer edits for a clinical database field related to a lab value for glucose in urine, you should design the database program so that the computer will not accept a number beyond a specified range of numbers.

    a. true
    b. false

11. A database inventory should be done when planning acquisition of a new computer system.

    a. true
    b. false

12. Since the location of care in a home health agency is in the patient's home, the nurse or therapist should bring the original record with him during the home visit.

    a. true
    b. false

CHAPTER REVIEW

Directions:

1. Tear out a Chapter Review Answer Sheet from the back of this review manual.

2. Read each question carefully before selecting an answer.

3. Write the correct or best answer on the answer sheet.

4. Answer all the questions since there is no penalty in this chapter review.

5. Check your answers with the answer key located at the end of this chapter review.

1. A physician is interested in knowing the case mix of his patients over the past year to be shared with a prospective partner. You produce the report using:

    a. unique patient count
    b. duplicated patient count
    c. primary health data
    d. truncated data

2. Which of the following would be of concern in qualitative analysis of the patient record?

    a. presence of the principal diagnosis and its authentication
    b. gaps in handwritten documentation such as nurses notes
    c. the record's reflection of the progression of care
    d. correct patient identification on every form

DELINQUENT CHART REPORT

Doctor	Charts Missing H&P's	Charts Missing Op Report	Charts Missing Signatures	Charts with Other Defic.	Total Charts
Green	4	1	23	1	25
Smith	1	4	2	5	6
Jones	8	—	14	3	16
Ames	—	3	9	15	28
Morgan	1	—	—	2	3

Rocky Mountain Hospital has an average of 344 discharges and an average of 178 operative procedures per month. Above is the delinquent chart report for the end of the month.

$$\frac{14}{344} = 4.07 \qquad \frac{8}{178} = 4.49$$

3. Referring to the report above, the hospital will receive a Type I deficiency due to:

    a. too many missing signatures
    b. too many missing operative reports
    c. too many charts incomplete
    d. too many missing histories and physicals

Latte Medical Center has an average of 988 discharges per month and 341 operations. They have 183 delinquent records. They have 17 missing histories and physicals. They have 5 missing operative reports. What kind of deficiencies do they have?

a. they have a Type I deficiency in histories and physicals
b. they have a Type I deficiency in operative reports
c. they have a Type I deficiency in the number of delinquent charts
d. they have no Type I deficiencies

The following information from a patient record was entered into the computer: Patient name is Anna Schleffenburg-Myerson, chart number 10/14/36, birth date 03-23-36, admitted 12-13-93 by Dr. Thomas Rocky. After data entry, the automated MPI data was reviewed as follows:

Master Patient Index Screen

Last Name	First Name	Chart Number
Schleffenburg-My	Anna	10/14/36

Birth date	Adm Date	MD Code	Physician
23-Mar-36	13-Dec-93	103A	Rocky, T

5. Referring to the information in the table above, which is an example of data that are *truncated* in a field?

a. 10/14/36
b. Schleffenburg-My
c. 13 Dec 93
d. 103A

6. Which allows many applications and many fields using relational tables of information?

a. file management system
b. flat file
c. database management system
d. application system

7. A health resources management committee made up of representatives of many departments can provide a number of information systems functions. Which is *not* a purpose of this committee?

a. act as an impartial "jury" to determine which department's computer needs should be met —to help overcome "turf wars
b. provide daily supervision of the data processing staff in the hiring, firing, and disciplining of employees
c. recommend elimination of manual systems that duplicate computer systems that are in place
d. approve the types of routine reports that will be generated by the computer and distributed to departments

The following are several types of data commonly found in the health information setting. Label each statement below according to the appropriate category they represent. When two possible categories exist, select the "best":

a. Numeric/integer
b. Text/character/category
c. Memo
d. Date
e. Time
f. Logic

_____a_____ 8. 220/110 [blood pressure field]

_____c_____ 9. History of Present Illness: This is a 50-year-old female who has complained of chest pain for the past 2 weeks and now enters for tests to rule out possible myocardial infarction.

_____b_____ 10. 250.10, 410.9 [ICD-9-CM code field]

_____a_____ 11. 17 [age field]

_____b_____ 12. Smith [attending physician field]

_____a_____ 13. $23.50 [value of the charge for xeroxing copies of chart]

_____X_____ 14. Has the physician been notified of the incident? (Yes/No)

Following is a computer coding scheme for type of re-questor for a release of information computer log at the correspondence desk.

```
┌─────────────────────────────────────┐
│ Type of Requestor                    │
│                                      │
│ 1 = Patient                          │
│ 2 = Third party payer                │
│ 3 = Attorney                         │
│ 4 = Physician                        │
│ 5 = Other health care provider       │
└─────────────────────────────────────┘
```

15. Referring to the information in the coding scheme above, is the coding scheme complete?

    a. Yes
    b. No

16. Identify an error in the following coding scheme for race/ethnicity of patient.

```
┌─────────────────────────────────────┐
│ Race/Ethnicity                       │
│                                      │
│ 1 = White                            │
│ 2 = Black                            │
│ 3 = Asian                            │
│ 4 = Spanish/American                 │
│ 5 = Jewish                           │
│ 6 = American Indian                  │
│ 7 = Other                            │
└─────────────────────────────────────┘
```

DISCHARGE SUMMARY

Patient: Peter N. Smith   00-14-92   Room: 316.2

This 50-year-old man was admitted to the hospital on December 29, 1991 in a state of acute hyperactivity. He laughed and joked freely, exhibited flight of ideas, with no evidence of hallucinations or deliusions. He has had a history of previous similar episodes dating back to 1963.

He was treated with electric shock therapy and phenothiazines, gradually improved and after eight shock treatments appeared dull, vacant and confused. He was then switched to sleep therapy with sodium amytal, remained confused for the next several days. Gradually his memory improved. Then his mood became one of depression. This was treated with psycho-therapy and antidepressant medications. He was discharged on January 26, 1992.

Final diagnosis: Manic-depressive illness, manic phase.

_____

John James, M.D.

17, 18, 19.

Referring to the discharge summary above, iden-tify general data elements missing from the report which are required by the JCAHO standards. Do *not* include the fact that the summary was not signed.

ROCKY MOUNTAIN HOSPITAL

BED CAPACITY AND PATIENT LISTING AS OF JANUARY 15 (11.59 P.M.)

2-NORTH

200	Alan Green
201	
202-1	Julie Chamberlain
202-2	Carol Edwards
202-3	Amber Mitchell
202-4	
203	William Morgan
204	
205	Ross Pierce
206	
207	
208	Carol Stevenson
209	
210	
211-1	
211-2	Michael Cline
212-1	Donna James
212-2	Tammy Sells
213-1	Patricia Murphy
213-2	Agnes Brown
213-3	
213-4	

2-SOUTH

220-1	
220-2	Lynn Redmond
220-3	Janice Bergan
220-4	Mary Jane Brady
220-5	
220-6	Diana Reely
221-1	Raymond Morris
221-2	Lloyd Jones
221-3	
221-4	

3-SOUTH

320-1	Angela Warren
320-2	Sue Oros
320-3	
320-4	
320-5	
320-6	
321-1	Henry Wilson
321-2	Lawrence Mills
321-3	Peter Ames
321-4	

3-NORTH

300	Alfred Clinton	307-1	John Henry
301		307-2	Barry Henderson
302-1	Mary Hinderberg	308	Mona Feinstein
302-2	Eileen Murphy	309-1	George Casey
303-1		309-2	William Chang
303-2	Nancy Allen	309-3	Neil Dawson
304		309-4	Daniel Quinsey
305	Sue McConaghy	310-1	
306-1		310-2	
306-2		311	

ROCKY MOUNTAIN HOSPITAL

ADMISSIONS, DISCHARGES, TRANSFERS

DATE: JANUARY 16 (11:59 P.M.)

ADMISSIONS		Adm. Date
303-2	Nancy Allen	1-16
320-3	Tina Leggett	1-16
320-4	Jean Lever	1-16
213-3	Willa Moore	1-16
204	Edward Reyes	1-16
309-4	Norman Schwab	1-16
213-2	Celest Sorensen	1-16
211-1	Sylvester Sykes	1-16
206	Thomas Young	1-16

DISCHARGES		Adm. Date	Disch. Date
220-4	Mary Jane Brady	12-29	1-16
321-2	Lawrence Mills	1-3	1-16
309-4	Daniel Quinsey	1-10	1-16
213-3	Michelle Ramsey	1-16	1-16
220-2	Lynn Redmond	1-8	1-16
206	Thomas Young	1-16	1-16

Transfers	From (old bed)	To (new bed)
Agnes Brown	213-2	310-1
Sue McConaghy	305	220-5
Amber Mitchell	202-3	321-4
Eileen Murphy	302-2	301
Sue Oros	320-2	302-2
Diana Reely	220-6	206

20, 21.
Referring to the information in the table on the previous page, what are the 2 errors on the ADT List?

The following information system was set up for a college's dental hygiene program-clinic in which they wanted to track information about individual patients as well as student activity as it related to the treatment of these patients. The following three tables were incorporated into the database:

PATIENT

Patient Number
Patient Last Name
Patient First Name
Patient Address
Patient City
Patient State
Patient Zip
Patient Birthdate

STUDENT

Student Number
Student Last Name
Student First Name
Student Address
Student City
Student State
Student Zip
Student Telephone Number
Date of College Admission
Date of Graduation

VISIT
Patient Number
Date of Visit
Calculus Classification Code
Gum Disease Code
Treatment Code
Student Number

---

22. Referring to the information in the tables above, what is the linking field between the VISIT TABLE and the STUDENT TABLE?

23. Referring to the information in the tables above, what is the linking field between the VISIT TABLE and the PATIENT table?

24. Which one of the following activities is appropriate for the health care organization's information resources management committee?

a. determine which quality assessment and improvement (QAI) software package to purchase
b. do the programming for a tumor registry application
c. design the computer screen for data entry of patient registration.
d. troubleshoot and fix computer equipment problems

25. Which is the concept of data quality that indicates that information is consistent, no matter how many times the same data is collected and entered into the system?

a. meaning
b. accessibility
c. reliability
d. validity

26. Which of the following data entries would be most difficult to complete and require the most instructions?

a. reimbursement type
b. cell type of cancer, based on information in the pathology report
c. next of kin
d. physical examination

27. Which is *not* included in a data dictionary?

a. type of field and width of each data item/column
b. a listing of the reports on which the data element appears
c. lists of all patients in the database
d. security levels for the field

28. Which is the *best* description of parallel process-ing?

    a. performing an activity both manually and electronically
    b. performing an application both the old way and with the newly installed computer system
    c. keeping redundant data on separate file management systems in two or more departments
    d. downloading data from the mainframe to a department terminal and uploading the data when complete

29. Which is *not* an appropriate security measure to prevent the corruption of data by the malicious intent of employees or ex-employees?

    a. change the password immediately upon employee termination
    b. print and review exception reports of audit trails of computer transactions
    c. have the computer immediately prohibit further access to any employee who fails to use the proper password the first time
    d. lock out any unauthorized employee accessing the computer after hours

30. It is recommended that report validation be performed:

    a. when ordered by the hospital administrator
    b. when a new data processing supervisor is hired
    c. on all reports before they are used
    d. on each type of report at the end of the year

31. Which is *not* an important feature of PC database software for a health information system?

    a. can set up user menus
    b. can set up own screen formats for data input
    c. can perform desk top publishing functions
    d. can import data from other databases

32. Which would be an effective method for controlling the confidentiality of computerized information by employees?

    a. detail written procedures for each application explaining precisely how to enter data into the system
    b. develop policies concerning data security that are supported by top level management
    c. acquire retinal scanning machine for each terminal
    d. require access to computerized information using fingerprint recognition

33. The Health Information Management Department plans to install an automated tumor registry. The vendor documentation is very lengthy giving instructions on how to work the system. All tumor registry staff think a "cheat sheet" or 1-2 page instruction summary should be written for ease of reference and for increasing data quality. Who should develop this reference tool?

    a. the HIM Department supervisor of that application
    b. one of the three employees who will perform that application
    c. the HIM Department director
    d. the Director of Information Systems

34. Which of the following statements demonstrates the principle of meaning as a data quality characteristic?

    a. the physician and patient should speak the same language when obtaining data at the point of service
    b. the home health record is available simultaneously to both the nurse and therapist treating the patient
    c. the patient's address is identical in both the master patient index and business office records
    d. on an average 1.2 scheduled patient appointments per day are no shows for Dr. Anderson

35. A _____ is a collection of stored information that can serve one or more computer applications, and which is independent of programs using the information.

36. The letter "Y" in a database represents:

    a. integer
    b. bit
    c. byte
    d. information

37. The numeral 2836 in a database represents:

    a. information
    b. datum
    c. byte
    d. file

38. The *patient's last name* in a database is stored in a:

    a. column
    b. row
    c. byte
    d. file

39. __redundancy__ is the term given to data that are entered over and over again in different application programs, e.g., patient name, address, social security number, telephone number, etc.

40. Which is a command-driven, standard industry sub-language designed to manipulate relational databases?

    a. SQL
    b. HL7
    c. Q7A
    d. R-ADT

41. According to the JCAHO, the clinical records of hospital discharged patients must be complete no later than:

    a. the day of discharge
    b. one week after discharge
    c. thirty days after discharge
    d. ninety days after discharge

42. Which is *not* related to the verification of the documentation's source?

    a. authorship
    b. authentication
    c. signature
    d. transcription

43. Duplicate storage media should be kept in:

    a. a room different from the one where the computer is located, but within the facility
    b. a building not housing the computer
    c. off-site storage
    d. either b or c

44. Documentation review for the electronic patient record would include:

    a. quantitative analysis
    b. qualitative analysis
    c. no content analysis since the computer can do this automatically
    d. none of the above

45. Which is a relational database management personal computer software?

    a. Lotus 1-2-3
    b. WordPerfect
    c. Paradox
    d. Pagemaker

46. Which of the following is *not* included in the Information Management standards of the JCAHO?

    a. library systems
    b. data processing activities
    c. health information management systems
    d. laboratory sample collection processes

47. Which position is *best* able to coordinate the information management activities in a health care facility?

    a. CEO
    b. CIO   *chief infor Organization*
    c. COO
    d. COS

48. What is the purpose of "clinical pertinence reviews" as required by the JCAHO?

    a. The quality of the documentation supports the diagnosis and treatment.
    b. Quality patient care was rendered to the patient.
    c. The x-rays or lab tests were appropriate for that disease condition.
    d. The software selected by the facility meets the needs of the medical staff.

PRETEST REVIEW ANSWER KEY

Directions:

1. Correct your Pretest Review Answer Sheet with the answers below by placing a slash (Example: 8) through the incorrect question number with a pen or pencil of a contrasting color.

2. Record the correct answer to the right of your answer on your answer sheet.

3. Record the total correct on the Initial Performance Grid in section four of this review manual.

4. Calculate your performance rate and also record on the grid.

5. Promptly locate the correct answer for each question missed in the chapter of the textbook.

6. Proceed to the chapter review if your performance rate was 80% or higher, otherwise, return to the chapter for further study.

1.	a	5.	a	9.	a
2.	b	6.	a	10.	b
3.	a	7.	b	11.	b
4.	b	8.	b	12.	b

CHAPTER REVIEW ANSWER KEY

Directions:

1. Correct your Chapter Review Answer Sheet with the answers below by placing a slash (Example: 8) through the incorrect question number with a pen or pencil of a contrasting color.

2. Record the correct answer to the right of your answer on your answer sheet.

3. Record the total correct on the Initial Performance Grid in section four of this review manual.

4. Calculate your performance rate and also record on the grid.

5. Promptly locate the correct answer for each question missed in the chapter of the textbook.

6. Proceed to the next assigned chapter in your study.

1.	a	6.	c	11.	a
2.	c	7.	b	12.	b
3.	d	8.	a	13.	a
4.	d	9.	c	14.	f—yes/no since not all database software have logic fields; b (text/category) could also be detected
5.	b	10.	b		

15. b - should have "other" category for miscellaneous requestors not on this list, such as family members, government agencies (not related to reimbursement)

16. (Any one) Code 5—religious preference; patient can be classified in more than one category: both white and spanish; both black and Jewish

17. significant findings

18. patient's condition on discharge

19. instructions to patient/family

20. Nancy Allen—is in bed 303-2 (11:59 pm, January 16) and then is listed as admitted on January 17 on the ADT list

21. Michelle Ramsey—is on the ADT (Discharge Section), but not in Admission Section: discharge entry notes this as an admittance/discharge on the same day

22. student number

23. patient number

24. a

25. c

26. d

27. c

28. b

29. c (should allow at least 3 tries)

30. c

31. c

32. b

33. a

34. d

35. database

36. c

37. b

38. a

39. redundancy

40. a

41. c

42. d

43. d

44. b

45. c (Lotus & WordPerfect have a file Manager/flat file)

46. d

47. b

48. a

DATA ACCESS AND RETENTION

6

PRETEST REVIEW

Directions:

1. Tear out a Pretest Review Answer Sheet from the back of this review manual.

2. Read each question carefully before selecting an answer.

3. Write the correct or best answer on the answer sheet.

4. Answer all the questions, since there is no penalty for this pretest review.

5. Check your answers with the answer key located near the end of this chapter.

1. The Master Patient Index contains information on inpatients and outpatients.

    a. True
    b. False

2. In a terminal digit filing system, if the number is 64-79-36, the tertiary number is 64.

    a. True
    b. False

3. Scanners are equipment devices basic to optical image processing.

    a. True
    b. False

4. When the destruction of health records is considered, the governing board should authorize approval.

    a. True
    b. False

5. To assure that the system will always be available, the optical imaging retrieval workstation should not be capable of running other software.

    a. True
    b. False

6. If a retention schedule is correctly followed, all records can be destroyed after 5 years.

    a. True
    b. False

7. An alphabetic identification system can only be used with an alphabetic filing methodology.

    a. True
    b. False

8. The legality of microfilm is questionable and should be investigated separately in each state.

    a. True
    b. False

computer output Microfilm

9. Records become inactive when the patient expires.

    a. True
    b. False

10. Transfer notices in a permanent filing system have a lower work priority than the retrieval of patient records from the file.

    a. True
    b. False

11. COM is a non-computerized micrographics storage option.

    a. True
    b. False

12. The patient address is a minimum data requirement in the Master Patient Index.

    a. True
    b. False

CHAPTER REVIEW

Directions:

1.   Tear out a Chapter Review Answer Sheet from the back of this review manual.

2.   Read each question carefully before selecting an answer.

3.   Write the correct or best answer on the answer sheet.

4.   Answer all the questions since there is no penalty in this chapter review.

5.   Check your answers with the answer key located at the end of this chapter review.

1.   In the process of destroying health records, the destruction schedule and plan should first be approved by the facility's administration.

   a.   True
   b.   False

2.   Programs and data files shared by users in a LAN are stored in a jukebox.

   a.   True
   b.   False

3.   Bar code symbology could be useful in tracking patients in Admitting Services, Social Services and Dietary Services, for example.

   a.   True
   b.   False

Match the abbreviations in the left column with the correct descriptor in the right column. Not all descriptors may have answers.

_c_	4. WORM	a.	a retrieval system that is computerized
_i_	5. UPS	b.	character representations in electronic storage
_k_	6. RAM	c.	a method of recording data on an optical disk
_h_	7. OCR	d.	the automatic transfer of computerized data to a laser disk
_j_	8. MSEC	e.	the process of transferring computerized data to microfilm
_b_	9. MB	f.	the computer-to-computer exchange of information based on standards
_g_	10. LAN	g.	a communications network linking various hardware devices within a location
_f_	11. EDI	h.	the machine recognition of printed characters
_e_	12. COM	i.	a device used to keep a system running during power failure
_d_	13. COLD	j.	expresses speed of electronic transactions
		k.	an expression for the main memory of a computer system
		l.	expresses the resolution of output material

Master Patient Index Screen

Name: Smith, John James   MR#: 12-34-56

DOB: 06-03-1936   SS#: 294-55-3235

Sex: M

Dates of Admission: 01-10-84   Discharge: 01-15-84
06-05-91   06-07-91
10-20-94   10-26-94

14. Referring to the information in the illustration above, what was the date of Mr. Smith's first admission?

    01-10-84

15. Referring to the information in the illustration above, on what day was Mr. Smith discharged on his last admission?

    26

16. Referring to the information in the illustration above, what is Mr. Smith's first name?

    John

17. Referring to the information in the illustration above, in what section of the terminal digit filing system would you begin to look for Mr. Smith's record?

    56 (terminal digit)

18. Referring to the information in the illustration above, in what month was Mr. Smith born?

    June

19. Optical disks are read by an electromagnetic head in the disk drive.

    a. True
    b.) False

20. The magnification ratio in microfilm is the inverse of the reduction ratio.

    a. True
    b. False

21. *space saving* is one advantage of implementing an optical imaging system.

22. A written description of a proposed system's concepts is a *System Summary*

23. An alphabetically-arranged database used for the location of patient records in a numeric identification system is called a *MPI*.

24. Bar code scanners must come in contact with a bar code label to read its contents.

    a. True
    b.) False

25. A centralized record management system provides more flexibility in file format for users than its decentralized alternative.

    a. True
    b.) False

26.) Bar code symbology code 39 has been approved for use in health care.

    a.) True
    b. False

27. An optical image system provides multi-user access to the same information.

    a. True
    b. False

28. Outguides aid in the correct placement of refiled records.

    a. True
    b. False

29. The patient date of birth is a minimum data requirement in the Master Patient Index.

    a. True
    b. False

30. A jukebox is a component of which system?

    a. optical imaging system
    b. CAR-roll microfilm system
    c. automated record tracking system
    d. computer output microfiche system

31. Which factor would be decreased by using cache memory in an optical imaging system?

    a. exchange time
    b. access time
    c. storage time
    d. video refresh rate

32. A file area that has limited space, low file activity and one primary file maintenance worker might benefit from choosing which type of filing equipment?

    a. open shelf filing units
    b. lateral filing cabinets
    c. vertical filing cabinets
    d. motorized revolving units

33. Which filing methodology would provide a high degree of accountability for filing accuracy, no backshifting, and highly accurate filing capability?

    a. terminal digit filing
    b. straight numeric filing
    c. alphabetic filing
    d. serial-unit filing

34. Using the terminal digit filing methodology, which number would be first in the file?

    a. 013291
    b. 911206
    c. 861971
    d. 165060

35. Which of the following is characteristic of an automated record tracking system?

    a. requisition slips are illegible
    b. workload is difficult to prioritize
    c. system is updated in real-time
    d. transfer notices are filed before patient records are retrieved

36. Why is the Master Patient Index maintained permanently?

    a. The Joint Commission on Accreditation of Healthcare Organizations requires that it be kept permanently.
    b. Patients cannot remember their number when asked for it.
    c. It does not occupy much space in comparison to maintaining the full record.
    d. Information in a numerical identification system cannot be located without it.

37. Which type of filming method must you choose to maintain the unit record concept and have the microfilm available where the patient is serviced?

    a. roll microfilm
    b. CAR-roll microfilm
    c. jacket microfilm
    d. CAR-jacket microfilm

38. A contracted microfilm service bureau usually quotes the price of their services as:

    a. the price per 1000 images
    b. the price per roll of film
    c. the hours of labor required
    d. the number of filing inches converted

39. To make a paper copy of a microfilm image, you use a:

    a. microfilm duplicator
    b. microfilm reader-printer
    c. microfilm developer
    d. contracted service bureau

40. When attempting to gain acceptance and purchase agreement for a new system, which document contains a written description of the system and an explanation of the system concepts?

    a. system diagram
    b. system summary
    c. financial summary
    d. implementation plan

41. Which abbreviation identifies the process of transferring data electronically from one computer system to another?

    a. COLD
    b. COM
    c. EDI
    d. ICR

42. The COM process most closely resembles which other process?

    a. WORM
    b. EDI
    c. COLD
    d. OCR

43. Which of the following is an indirect cost of a facility's storage and retrieval system?

    a. regular and temporary labor costs
    b. light and heat
    c. storage and supply costs
    d. equipment costs

44. Implementation of an imaged-based storage and retrieval system frees up high-priced floor space that could be put to better use. This is an example of:

    a. direct costs
    b. direct savings
    c. offsetting revenues
    d. indirect costs

45. Using the straight numeric filing methodology, which number would be first in the file?

    a. 62374
    b. 73912
    c. 12465
    d. 11320

46. Your file maintenance staff are having trouble locating the terminal digit sections quickly. To help them, you could add more:

    a. outcards
    b. outguides
    c. file guides
    d. file maintenance staff

47. Which filing equipment protects records against environmental damaged?

    a. open shelf files
    b. filing cabinets
    c. motorized revolving units
    d. compressible units

48. Which microfilm format can be color-coded and filed in a miniature version of the paper system?

    a. roll microfilm
    b. jacket microfilm
    c. CAR-roll microfilm
    d. CAR-jacket microfilm

PRETEST REVIEW ANSWER KEY

Directions:

1. Correct your Pretest Review Answer Sheet with the answers below by placing a slash (Example: 8) through the incorrect question number with a pen or pencil of a contrasting color.

2. Record the correct answer to the right of your answer on your answer sheet.

3. Record the total correct on the Initial Performance Grid in section four of this review manual.

4. Calculate your performance rate and also record on the grid.

5. Promptly locate the correct answer for each question missed in the chapter of the textbook.

6. Proceed to the chapter review if your performance rate was 80% or higher, otherwise, return to the chapter for further study.

1.	a	5.	b	9.	b
2.	a	6.	b	10.	b
3.	a	7.	b	11.	b
4.	a	8.	b	12.	b

CHAPTER REVIEW ANSWER KEY

Directions:

1. Correct your Chapter Review Answer Sheet with the answers below by placing a slash (Example: 8) through the incorrect question number with a pen or pencil of a contrasting color.

2. Record the correct answer to the right of your answer on your answer sheet.

3. Record the total correct on the Initial Performance Grid in section four of this review manual.

4. Calculate your performance rate and also record on the grid.

5. Promptly locate the correct answer for each question missed in the chapter of the textbook.

6. Proceed to the next assigned chapter in your study.

1.	a	6.	k	11.	f
2.	b	7.	h	12.	e
3.	a	8.	j	13.	d
4.	c	9.	b	14.	01-10-84
5.	i	10.	g	15.	26th

16.	John	26.	a	38.	a
17.	56	27.	a	39.	b
18.	6th month or June	28.	a	40.	b
19.	b	29.	a	41.	c
20.	a	30.	a	42.	c
21.	(any one) space savings; productivity gains; multi-user access; system security & control; or retrieval of information	31.	b	43.	b
		32.	d	44.	c
		33.	a	45.	d
22.	System Summary	34.	b	46.	c
23.	Master Patient Index (MPI)	35.	c	47.	b
24.	b	36.	d	48.	b
25.	b	37.	c		

CODING AND CLASSIFICATION SYSTEMS

7

PRETEST REVIEW

Directions:

1. Tear out a Pretest Review Answer Sheet from the back of this review manual.

2. Read each question carefully before selecting an answer.

3. Write the correct or best answer on the answer sheet.

4. Answer all the questions, since there is no penalty for this pretest review.

5. Check your answers with the answer key located near the end of this chapter.

1. In the APG reimbursement system, if patients are assigned to more than one APG, a bundling process is necessitated to determine the payment.

    a. True
    b. False

2. Comorbidities can be found on the history and physical examination record.

    a. True
    b. False

3. DRGs are a prospective case mix payment mechanism for inpatients.

    a. True
    b. False

4. A complication is a condition which is present at admission.

    a. True
    b. False

5. The assignment of a DRG is based on the principal diagnosis and significant operating room procedure, if there was a procedure.

    a. True
    b. False

6. An encoder is used to divide patients into DRGs.

    a. True
    b. False

7. ICD-9-CM is used in hospitals and physician offices.

    a. True
    b. False

8. HCPCS and CPT are classification systems.

    a. True
    b. False

9. Malpractice insurance expense is taken into consideration in the relative value units of the RBRVS system.

   a. True
   b. False

10. The UHDDS captures data on hospital inpatients.

    a. True
    b. False

11. CPT codes are Level 1 codes.

    a. True
    b. False

12. APGs are like DRGs and are based on the HCPCS code.

    a. True
    b. False

CHAPTER REVIEW

Directions:

1. Tear out a Chapter Review Answer Sheet from the back of this review manual.

2. Read each question carefully before selecting an answer.

3. Write the correct or best answer on the answer sheet.

4. Answer all the questions since there is no penalty in this chapter review.

5. Check your answers with the answer key located at the end of this chapter review.

1. Name the form for billing federally-funded inpatients for hospital services.

2. HCPCS is used for coding diagnoses.

    a. True
    b. False

3. Sequencing codes is a processing task associated with a valid coding process.

    a. True
    b. False

4. Maximizing reimbursement is unethical if it cannot be verified by the content of the patient record.

    a. True
    b. False

5. DSM-IIIR is used in:

    a. long term care facilities
    b. psychiatric hospitals
    c. HMO's and PPO's
    d. psychiatrist offices

6. Codes such as: T-xy300, M-40000, D-6501, E2300 are examples of what kind of codes?

    a. CPT
    b. ICD-9-CM
    c. HCPCS
    d. SNOMED

7. Which of the following is true?

    a. The PRO can change a principal diagnosis but cannot add diagnoses.
    b. The PRO can alter a diagnosis which cannot be verified by the content of the record.
    c. The PRO can add a diagnosis that may change the DRG.
    d. Both a and b

8. HCPCS/CPT and ICD-9-CM are the primary coding systems in use in health care today.

    a. True
    b. False

9. Coding can be performed concurrently or retrospectively to the patient's discharge.

    a. True
    b. False

10. One purpose for assigning a number to diagnoses and procedures is for retrieving the data efficiently.

    a. True
    b. False

11. You are a coding supervisor at Rocky Mountain Hospital and are trying to determine how many inpatient coders you need. You have approximately 1500 discharges including deaths per month and each coder will work 150 hours per month. It has been determined that coders should be allowed 20 minutes to code each record. How many coders do you need?

    a. 2.0
    b. 3.3
    c. 4.2
    d. 4.4

12. ICD-9-CM is used for coding death certificates in the U.S.

    a. True
    b. False

13. ICD-9-CM is a world-wide classification system which is revised every 10 years by the WHO.

    a. True
    b. False

Match the abbreviations in the left column with the correct descriptor in the right column. Not all descriptors may have answers.

_____ 14. APACHE

_____ 15. CPT

_____ 16. DSM

_____ 17. HCPCS

_____ 18. ICD-9-CM

_____ 19. ICD-O

_____ 20. RBRVS

_____ 21. SNOMED

_____ 22. UB-92

_____ 23. UHDDS

a. classification

b. data set

c. nomenclature

d. reimbursement form

e. severity of illness system

f. reimbursement method

24. The Central Office on ICD9-CM is located with the:

    a. AHA
    b. AHIMA
    c. HCFA
    d. NCHS

25. Which is *not* descriptive of Level l codes in the HCPCS?

    a. Level l codes are CPT codes
    b. Level l codes are published every two years
    c. Level l codes are numeric
    d. Level l codes are strictly for physician services

26. The PRO review process is used for all inpatients.

    a. True
    b. False

27. Reliability and completeness are factors associated with the quality of coded data.

    a. True
    b. False

28. The number of coders needed to code inpatient cases can be calculated to ensure the workload is handled. The numerator for this equation would be:

    a. total number of records to be coded x number of discharges for the period
    b. number of hours worked per coder for the time period
    c. mean coding time per record x number of discharges and deaths for period
    d. coding time per record x number of discharges for the period

29. The quality of coded data can be assessed in one way from the disease and operation indexes by employing criteria.

    a. True
    b. False

30. E codes and V codes can be used to code principal diagnoses.

    a. True
    b. False

31. Supplemental resources for ICD-9-CM coders in inpatient facilities should include:

    a. encoders
    b. *Coding Clinic*
    c. *CPT Assistant*
    d. both a and b

32. Concurrent coding is performed at the same time as discharge abstracting.

    a. True
    b. False

PRO DRG VALIDATION PROCESS

- **Accuracy of coding the principal diagnosis, secondary diagnosis and procedure codes**

- **Accuracy of codes on UB-92**

- **Accuracy of discharge disposition**

---

33. A grouper assigns a DRG based on age, sex, principal diagnosis and comorbidities.

    a. True
    b. False

34. Coding a cerebral concussion, only, when the temporal bone was also fractured is a reliability problem.

    a. True
    b. False

35. Referring to the information in the table above, what validation item is missing from the PRO DRG validation process?

36. The intent of severity of illness classification systems is improved reliability and validity of patient care cost predictions.

    a. True
    b. False

37.   Which is *not* a severity of illness coding system?

 a.   ATLAS
 b.   APACHE
 c.   RBRVS
 d.   SNOMED

38.   There are both medical and surgical DRGs.

 a.   True
 b.   False

39.   DRGs and APGs are affected by:

 a.   E codes
 b.   V codes
 c.   procedure codes
 d.   all of the above

40.   Which coding system is associated with "unbun-dling?"

 a.   ICD-9-CM
 b.   CPT
 c.   HCPCS
 d.   none of the above

41.   Classification systems include the systematic list-ing of proper names for diagnoses and procedures.

 a.   True
 b.   False

42.   Classifications and nomenclatures use both alpha and numeric characters.

 a.   True
 b.   False

43.   Sequencing diagnosis codes is a function required for UHDDS abstracting.

 a.   True
 b.   False

44.   Which diagnosis should be listed first when se-quencing codes?

 a.   principal diagnosis
 b.   primary diagnosis
 c.   significant diagnosis
 d.   secondary diagnosis

45.   Which of the following would *not* require HCPCS/ CPT codes?

 a.   patient office visit
 b.   hospital ambulatory surgery visit
 c.   hospital inpatient visit
 d.   hospital outpatient visit

46.   ICD-9-CM and HCPCS codes are assigned relative values for Medicare reimbursement purposes.

 a.   True
 b.   False

47.   DRG optimization is ordinarily *not* affected by the coding of complications and comorbidities.

 a.   True
 b.   False

48.   Which is *excluded* from ICD-O codes?

 a.   behavior
 b.   etiology
 c.   morphology
 d.   topography

PRETEST REVIEW ANSWER KEY

Directions:

1. Correct your Pretest Review Answer Sheet with the answers below by placing a slash (Example: 8̸) through the incorrect question number with a pen or pencil of a contrasting color.

2. Record the correct answer to the right of your answer on your answer sheet.

3. Record the total correct on the Initial Performance Grid in section four of this review manual.

4. Calculate your performance rate and also record on the grid.

5. Promptly locate the correct answer for each question missed in the chapter of the textbook.

6. Proceed to the chapter review if your performance rate was 80% or higher, otherwise, return to the chapter for further study.

1.	a	5.	b	9.	a
2.	a	6.	b	10.	a
3.	a	7.	a	11.	a
4.	b	8.	a	12.	b

CHAPTER REVIEW ANSWER KEY

Directions:

1. Correct your Chapter Review Answer Sheet with the answers below by placing a slash (Example: 8̸) through the incorrect question number with a pen or pencil of a contrasting color.

2. Record the correct answer to the right of your answer on your answer sheet.

3. Record the total correct on the Initial Performance Grid in section four of this review manual.

4. Calculate your performance rate and also record on the grid.

5. Promptly locate the correct answer for each question missed in the chapter of the textbook.

6. Proceed to the next assigned chapter in your study.

1.	UB-92	6.	d	11.	b(1500 x .33)/150
2.	b	7.	c	12.	b
3.	a	8.	a	13.	b
4.	a	9.	a	14.	e
5.	b	10.	a	15.	a

16.	a	27.	a	38.	a
17.	a	28.	d	39.	c
18.	a	29.	a	40.	b
19.	a	30.	b	41.	b
20.	f	31.	d	42.	a
21.	c	32.	b	43.	a
22.	d	33.	b	44.	a
23.	b	34.	b	45.	c
24.	a	35.	accuracy of sequencing	46.	b
25.	b	36.	a	47.	b
26.	b	37.	d	48.	b

REGISTRIES 8

PRETEST REVIEW

Directions:

1. Tear out a Pretest Review Answer Sheet from the back of this review manual.

2. Read each question carefully before selecting an answer.

3. Write the correct or best answer on the answer sheet.

4. Answer all the questions, since there is no penalty for this pretest review.

5. Check your answers with the answer key located near the end of this chapter.

1. An annual report is required of cancer registry programs approved by the ACS.

    a. True
    b. False

2. Trauma registries may be hospital or population-based.

    a. True
    b. False

3. A casefinding source for a hospital cancer registry includes pathology reports, for example, bone marrow, hematology and cytology reports.

    a. True
    b. False

4. A casefinding source for a hospital cancer registry includes the disease index.

    a. True
    b. False

5. ICD-O-2 permits coding of neoplastic tissue grades.

    a. True
    b. False

6. A cancer request log should contain the purpose or use of data from each individual requesting data.

    a. True
    b. False

7. A cancer request log should contain the authorization for release of data.

    a. True
    b. False

8. The categories of cancer registries are generally defined as hospital or population-based.

    a. True
    b. False

9.   The American College of Surgeons approved hospital cancer programs are limited to single facility, acute care hospital programs.

     a.   True
     b.   False

10. The American College of Surgeons requires the cancer committee of a hospital-based cancer registry to meet at least twice a year.

     a.   True
     b.   False

11. The purpose of a birth defects registry is determined by the type of case ascertainment system it operates.

     a.   True
     b.   False

12. The Injury Severity Scale is required of trauma registries by the American College of Surgeons.

     a.   True
     b.   False

CHAPTER REVIEW

Directions:

1. Tear out a Chapter Review —Answer Sheet from the back of this review manual.

2. Read each question carefully before selecting an answer.

3. Write the correct or best answer on the answer sheet.

4. Answer all the questions since there is no penalty in this chapter review.

5. Check your answers with the answer key located at the end of this chapter review.

ACCESSION REGISTER				
Acc. #	Patient's Name	Primary Site	Site #	Date of Diagnosis
94-0001/00	Raggedy, A	Liver	C22	01/02/94
94-0002/02	Possum, M.	Colon	C18	01/03/94
93-0345/02	Cake, P.	Lung	C34	01/03/94
94-0004/01	Doe, John	Prostate	C61	01/04/94
94/0004/02	Doe, John	Colon	C18	01/04/94
94/0006/00	Lincoln, M.	Breast	C50	01/04/94

1. Referring to the data in the illustration above, Raggedy, A's tumor was not malignant as noted by the accession number.

    a. True
    b. False

2. Referring to the data in the illustration above, P. Cake was first diagnosed with cancer at this hospital in 1993.

    a. True
    b. False

3. Referring to the data in the illustration above, there are 6 different patients—1 female and 5 males.

    a. True
    b. False

4. Referring to the data in the illustration above, Acc.# 94-0002/02 means this is the patient's second admission with cancer.

    a. True
    b. False

5. Referring to the data in the illustration above, how many case have only one primary tumor?

Match the terms in the left column with a correct descriptor in the right column. Not all descriptors may have an answer.

_____ 6. differentiation

_____ 7. etiology

_____ 8. morphology

_____ 9. reference date

_____ 10. surveillance

_____ 11. topography

_____ 12. staging

_____ 13. grade

_____ 14. histology

_____ 15. follow-up

a. system for documenting the extent or spread of cancer

b. site of origin of a neoplasm

c. designates the degree of differentiation

d. the beginning point of data collection by a registry

e. the monitoring of incidence and trends associated with a disease

f. the cause or origin of a disease process

g. the structure, composition and function of a tissue

h. the form and structure of an organ or part

i. continued medical surveillance of a case

j. case that meets criteria for inclusion in a database

k. the degree to which a tumor resembles normal tissue

l. number of new cases for a period

16. A casefinding source for a hospital cancer registry includes the Oncology Unit log.

   a. True
   b. False

17. A casefinding source for a hospital cancer registry includes the Radiation Therapy department log.

   a. True
   b. False

18. ICD-O-2 permits coding of topography.

   a. True
   b. False

19. ICD-O-2 permits coding of differentiation.

   a. True
   b. False

20. A cancer registry request log should contain the date of request and the name of the individual requesting data.

   a. True
   b. False

21. A cancer registry log should contain the topic of reports using cancer data and the time period covered by the report.

   a. True
   b. False

22. A cancer registry log should contain the list of patients included in any reports.

   a. True
   b. False

23. A cancer registry log should contain the final disposition of the data requested.

   a. True
   b. False

24. Cancer registries have been established to:

    a. investigate the cause(s) of cancer as a disease
    b. eradicate cancer as a disease
    c. assess cancer incidence, treatment and end results
    d. monitor physician performance in treating cancer patients

25. The National Cancer Institute's SEER Program operates population-based cancer registries covering approximately _____ percent of the U.S. population.

    a. 3%
    b. 13%
    c. 23%
    d. 33%

26. The primary goal of hospital-based cancer registries is to:

    a. improve the care of the patient with cancer
    b. monitor local cancer incidence and trends
    c. conduct basic cancer research
    d. assess hospital costs associated with cancer patients

27. Which of the following is *not* a required component of an approved hospital cancer program?

    a. cancer committee
    b. cancer registry
    c. cancer conferences
    d. cancer control

28. The reference date for a cancer registry is defined as the date the:

    a. registry is implemented
    b. data collection begins
    c. cancer committee is formed
    d. cancer program is approved

29. Which is an objective of population-based cancer registries?

    a. efficacy of treatment
    b. cancer incidence surveillance
    c. cancer control
    d. patient follow up

30. Which is *not* a purpose of a trauma registry?

    a. track patient survival
    b. improve pre-and-post hospital care
    c. provide descriptive epidemiology
    d. evaluate program and management

31. Which of the following cancer registry files is considered a temporary file?

    a. accession register
    b. follow-up
    c. patient index
    d. primary site

32. Which of the following is intended to assess the annual caseload and provide each patient with a registry identification number?

    a. accession register
    b. follow-up
    c. patient index
    d. primary site

33. A cancer patient, first seen in 1994 with colon cancer and who had a history of breast cancer, would be assigned which of the following numbers?

    a. 94-0001/00
    b. 94-0001/01
    c. 94-0001/02
    d. 94-0000/01

34. What is the maximum delay permissable in an approved hospital cancer program for case abstracting after the date of the patient's initial diagnosis?

    a. one month
    b. three months
    c. six months
    d. twelve months

35. The American College of Surgeons places accountability for quality control of registry data with the:

    a. cancer registrar
    b. cancer committee
    c. quality assurance committee
    d. medical advisor to the cancer registry

36. Cancer registry computer software usually provides for which of the following:

    a. word processing
    b. statistical analysis
    c. patient care evaluation
    d. networking with hospital information systems

37. Which of the following cancer data may be released without patient authorization?

    a. aggregate
    b. patient
    c. physician
    d. facility

38. The American College of Surgeons requires _____ patient care evaluation study(ies) annually.

    a. one short term (process)
    b. one long term (outcome)
    c. one short term and one long term
    d. either a short term or a long term

39. The American College of Surgeons requires cancer conferences be held weekly or monthly depending on:

    a. the annual number of cancer cases seen
    b. the age of the cancer registry
    c. the services provided
    d. the cancer program category

40. Documentation for cancer conferences must include the following:

    a. recommendations for treatment
    b. copies of case protocols
    c. attendance sign-in sheet
    d. date of follow-up presentation

41. Which of the following organizations offers a national certification examination for cancer registry professionals?

    a. American Cancer Society
    b. American Health Information Management Association
    c. National Cancer Registrars Association
    d. North American Association of Central Cancer Registrars

42. AIDS registry data is available for use by all *but* the following?

    a. hospital administration and medical staff
    b. local and state health agencies
    c. community AIDS agencies
    d. Centers for Disease Control

43. AIDS cases are identified for inclusion in the registry database using the same casefinding sources used by cancer registries, plus:

    a. respiratory therapy departments
    b. pathology laboratories
    c. health information departments
    d. oncology units

44. Birth Defects surveillance systems are characterized as:

    a. rapid case ascertainment systems only
    b. active case ascertainment systems only
    c. passive case ascertainment systems only
    d. active or passive case ascertainment systems

45. Hospital-based disease registries include all but which of the following?

    a. AIDS
    b. birth defects
    c. implant
    d. trauma

46. Which of the following is *not* a case criterion for a trauma registry?

    a. admission to the hospital for 48 hours
    b. ICD-9-CM Injury Code between 800 and 959.9
    c. admission to an operating room or intensive care unit
    d. death in the hospital emergency room.

47. ICD-O-2 permits coding of neoplastic morphology.

    a. True
    b. False

48. Trauma registries use only ICD-9-CM injury and E codes.

    a. True
    b. False

PRETEST REVIEW ANSWER KEY

Directions:

1. Correct your Pretest Review Answer Sheet with the answers below by placing a slash (Example: 8) through the incorrect question number with a pen or pencil of a contrasting color.

2. Record the correct answer to the right of your answer on your answer sheet.

3. Record the total correct on the Initial Performance Grid in section four of this review manual.

4. Calculate your performance rate and also record on the grid.

5. Promptly locate the correct answer for each question missed in the chapter of the textbook.

6. Proceed to the chapter review if your performance rate was 80% or higher, otherwise, return to the chapter for further study.

1.	a	5.	a	9.	b
2.	a	6.	a	10.	b
3.	a	7.	b	11.	a
4.	a	8.	a	12.	b

CHAPTER REVIEW ANSWER KEY

Directions:

1. Correct your Chapter Review Answer Sheet with the answers below by placing a slash (Example: 8) through the incorrect question number with a pen or pencil of a contrasting color.

2. Record the correct answer to the right of your answer on your answer sheet.

3. Record the total correct on the Initial Performance Grid in section four of this review manual.

4. Calculate your performance rate and also record on the grid.

5. Promptly locate the correct answer for each question missed in the chapter of the textbook.

6. Proceed to the next assigned chapter in your study.

1.	b	6.	k	11.	b
2.	a	7.	f	12.	a
3.	b	8.	h	13.	c
4.	b	9.	d	14.	g
5.	2	10.	e	15.	i

16.	b	27.	d	38.	c
17.	a	28.	b	39.	d
18.	a	29.	b	40.	c
19.	a	30.	a	41.	c
20.	a	31.	b	42.	c
21.	a	32.	a	43.	a
22.	b	33.	c	44.	d
23.	a	34.	c	45.	c
24.	c	35.	b	46.	a
25.	b	36.	b	47.	a
26.	a	37.	a	48.	a

RESEARCH, STATISTICS AND EPIDEMIOLOGY 9

PRETEST REVIEW

Directions:

1. Tear out a Pretest Review Answer Sheet from the back of this review manual.

2. Read each question carefully before selecting an answer.

3. Write the correct or best answer on the answer sheet.

4. Answer all the questions, since there is no penalty for this pretest review.

5. Check your answers with the answer key located near the end of this chapter.

1. A graph that includes continuous interval categories on the X-axis is a histogram.

   a. True
   b. False

2. Ranked data are discrete data.

   a. True
   b. False

3. A bar graph displays the frequency of variables on the Y-axis.

   a. True
   b. False

4. The Y-axis is the horizontal axis.

   a. True
   b. False

5. A frequency distribution can be used to group ordinal data and their total number of observations.

   a. True
   b. False

6. The NCHS collects data on births, deaths and fetal deaths.

   a. True
   b. False

7. The numerical expression 10:1 is called a proportion.

   a. True
   b. False

8. 1 in 100,000 is an expression of a rate.

   a. True
   b. False

9. The anesthesia death rate can be referred to as a cause-specific death rate.

   a. True
   b. False

10. A death occurring within 48 hours after surgery is calculated in the post-operative death rate.

    a. True
    b. False

11. The denominator for the post-operative death rate is the total number of operative procedures for the period.

    a. True
    b. False

12. The null hypothesis is stated as if no differences between two groups exist.

    a. True
    b. False

CHAPTER REVIEW

Directions:

1. Tear out a Chapter Review Answer Sheet from the back of this review manual.

2. Read each question carefully before selecting an answer.

3. Write the correct or best answer on the answer sheet.

4. Answer all the questions since there is no penalty in this chapter review.

5. Check your answers with the answer key located at the end of this chapter review.

ROCKY MOUNTAIN HOSPITAL

MONTHLY REPORT

July 1995	Hospital Statistics
Discharges (including deaths)	1099
Total Deaths:	55
Inpatient (incl. 2 coroners cases)	51
Outpatient	4
Total Autopsies:	11
Inpatient	10
Outpatient	1

1. Referring to the data in the report above, the net autopsy rate is:

   a. 19.6%
   b. 20.0%
   c. 20.4%
   d. 22.5%

2. Referring to the data in the report in the column on the left, the adjusted hospital autopsy rate is:

   a. 1.0%
   b. 18.9%
   c. 20.8%
   d. 22.1%

3. Nosocomial infections are those infections:

   a. occurring 72 hours after admission
   b. occurring less than 72 hours before admission
   c. occurring after surgery
   d. both a and c

4. The ———————— is the average number of observations.

5. The denominator for the net death rate is:

   a. total inpatient deaths less inpatient deaths less than 48 hours after admission x 100
   b. total inpatient deaths
   c. total discharges and deaths less inpatient deaths occurring within 48 hours of admission
   d. total discharges and deaths x 100

6. A whole number divided in 100 parts is a ————————.

7. The post-operative death rate is *not* considered a cause-specific death rate.

   a. True
   b. False

8. The post-operative death rate is calculated on the total number of deaths occurring within:

   a. 48 hours of surgery
   b. 3 days of surgery
   c. 10 days of surgery
   d. none of the above

9. If a p-value of .001 was obtained, the researcher would most likely:

   a. accept the null hypothesis
   b. reject the null hypothesis
   c. reject the alternative hypothesis
   d. none of the above

10. If a researcher accepts the null hypothesis when it is false, he has committed a type II error.

    a. True
    b. False

11. The——————————— denotes the middlemost value when the values are arranged in numerical order.

12. ————————————— is a measure of how often data are classified in the same manner.

Match the terms in the left column with the correct descriptor in the right column. Not all descriptors may have answers.

_____ 13. continuous data

_____ 14. discrete data

_____ 15. ordinal data

_____ 16. nominal data

_____ 17. confounding variable

_____ 18. dependent variable

_____ 19. independent variable

a. data that can assume a whole number such as number of sisters and brothers

b. data that can have an assigned numerical value such as race or sex

c. the variable under study

d. statistic demonstrating how values are spread around the mean

e. data that can assume an infinite number of possible values such as charges

f. variable having a relationship with the study variable

g. ranking of data according to a criterion

h. variable that can have an effect on the study variable and the characteristic under study

20. The _____ is the difference between the highest and lowest values.

21. Which is true regarding comorbidities?

    a. they are a pre-existing condition
    b. they generally increase the length of stay
    c. they affect mortality and morbidity rates
    d. all of the above

22. What was the median length of stay for these psychiatric patients: 4, 11, 2, 1, 8, 22, 7.

    a. 4 days
    b. 7 days
    c. 8 days
    d. none of the above

23. Referring to question #22, the range for these patients' length of stay was:

    a. 7
    b. 13
    c. 21
    d. none of the above

24. A researcher desires to estimate the relative risk an individual has of acquiring a disease to which he has been exposed. What statistic is appropriate for this purpose?

    a. incidence
    b. relative risk
    c. cohort study
    d. odds ratio

25. The _____ demonstrates how values are spread around the mean and is the square root of the variance.

26. Which variable is *not* related to the others?

    a. ranked
    b. categorical
    c. qualitative
    d. nominal

27. In Rocky Mountain High County, the number of teenage girls who had delivered a child was 2226. The population of teenage girls in this county was 110,000. The prevalence rate of teenage deliveries was:

    a. .02 or less than 1 case per 1000
    b. 2 cases per 1000
    c. 20 cases per 1000
    d. 200 cases per 1000

28. Referring to question #27, a pie chart displaying teenage deliveries would show that the prevalence rate or teen pregnancy data should occupy:

    a. 2 degrees
    b. 20 degrees
    c. 72 degrees
    d. none of the above

29. The 300 bed Rocky Mountain Hospital had a total of 2200 discharges (including deaths) and a total of 7,600 inpatient service days during the month of June. The percentage of occupancy was:

    a. 40.4%
    b. 84.4%
    c. 7,600:9,000
    d. 7,600:9,300

30. The average length of stay in the Intensive Care, Cardiac Care and Intermediate Care units were 13, 7 and 4 respectively. The three units have seen 18, 10 and 18 patients, respectively. What was the weighted average length of stay?

    a. 6.2 days
    b. 7.4 days
    c. 7.9 days
    d. 8.2 days

152 INPATIENTS IN ROCKY MOUNTAIN HOSPITAL

Total Charges ($)	Frequency	Relative Frequency (%)
0-4,999	62	40.8%
5,000-9,999	46	30.3%
10,000-14,999	25	——
15,000-19,999	7	4.6%
20,000-24,999	5	3.3%
25,000-29,999	4	2.6%
30,000-34,999	0	0
35,000-39,999	0	0
40,000-44,999	0	0
45,000-49,999	3	2.0%

31. Referring to the table above, what kind of data is shown?

32. Referring to the table above, what was the relative frequency for the data in the 10,000–14,999 interval?

ROCKY MOUNTAIN HOSPITAL ADMISSIONS BY RESIDENCE

September

	City n = 77 no. (%)	Suburbs n = 38 no. (%)	Rural n = 29 no. (%)	Total n = 144 no. (%)
Hospital A	20 (26%)	8 (21%)	12 (41%)	40 (28%)
Hospital B	30 (39%)	4 (11%)	9 (31%)	43 (30%)
Hospital C	10 (13%)	12 (32%)	6 (21%)	28 (19%)
Hospital D	17 (22%)	14 (37%)	2 (7%)	33 (23%)
Totals	77 (100%)	38 (100%)	29 (100%)	144 (100%)

33. Referring to the table immediately above, what kind of data is shown?

34. Referring to the table immediately above, which hospital appears to be located in the suburbs?

35. Referring to the table immediately above, which hospital drew the least patients from the city?

36. Referring to the table immediately above, which hospital had the fewest admissions for September?

STUDENT PERCEPTIONS OF LEADERSHIP CHARACTERISTICS

| | Management Clinical Internship | | | |
| | Before n = 35 | | After n = 35 | |
Leadership Characteristic Ranking	no.	%	no.	%
1 Very Weak	5	14%	0	0%
2 Weak	10	29%	1	3%
3 Moderate	15	43%	5	14%
4 Strong	2	6%	12	34%
5 Very Strong	3	9%	17	49%

37. Referring to the table immediately above, what kind of data is shown?

38. Referring to the table immediately above, it appears from the information that the leadership perceptions of the majority of students improved as a result of their clinical internship in management. Do you agree or disagree?
   a. yes
   b. no

PRINCIPAL HEALTH INSURANCE COVERAGE BY SEX

December

	Male n = 50 no. (%)	Female n = 50 no. (%)	Total n = 100 no. (%)
Medicare	13 (26%)	25 (50%)	38 (38%)
Medicaid	2 (4%)	6 (12%)	8 (8%)
Blue Cross	25 (50%)	10 (20%)	35 (35%)
Commercial	9 (18%)	6 (12%)	15 (15%)
Other	1 (2%)	3 (6%)	4 (4%)
Totals	50 (100%)	50 (100%)	100 (100%)

39. Referring to the table immediately above, what kind of data is shown?

40. Referring to the table immediately above, which fiscal agent provided more covered care for females than others?

LENGTH OF STAY (LOS)
PATIENTS WITH VIRAL PNEUMONIA

Community Acquired		Nosocomial	
MR#	LOS	MR#	LOS
207658	20	123579	15
214592	10	275816	22
221459	7	254137	18
158645	14	321096	10
129876	8	153992	8
Mean =	———	Mean =	———
Median =	———	Median =	———

41. Referring to the table immediately above, what was the mean LOS for patients having community-acquired viral pneumonia?

42. What was the median LOS for patients having nosocomial viral pneumonia?

43. Referring to the table immediately above, what data is missing for calculating the weighted mean?

INCIDENCE RATE OF CARDIOVASCULAR DISEASE

	Population	Cases	Incidence Rate
Exercise	1000	50	———
No Exercise	1000	145	———
Total	———	———	———

44. Referring to the table immediately above, what would be the numerator for calculating the incidence rate of cardiovascular disease in the study?

EXAMPLES OF STATISTICS

A	B	C	D
3 : 10,000	3/10,000 = 0.0003	0.03%	30 in 1000,000

45. Referring to the table immediately above, in which column is the ratio specified?

46. Once the birth or death certificate is complete, the original certificate is filed with the:

    a. NCHS
    b. National Death Index (NDI)
    c. state registrar
    d. local registrar

47. In the case-control study design, the cases are those individuals:

    a. with the disease under study
    b. without the disease under study
    c. with the health characteristic or risk factor under study
    d. without the health characteristic or risk factor under study

48. An experimental study in which an intervention or treatment is tested on a group or population in the community is called:

    a. clinical trial
    b. quality assessment study
    c. descriptive study
    d. community trial

PRETEST REVIEW ANSWER KEY

Directions:

1. Correct your Pretest Review Answer Sheet with the answers below by placing a slash (Example: ~~8~~) through the incorrect question number with a pen or pencil of a contrasting color.

2. Record the correct answer to the right of your answer on your answer sheet.

3. Record the total correct on the Initial Performance Grid in section four of this review manual.

4. Calculate your performance rate and also record on the grid.

5. Promptly locate the correct answer for each question missed in the chapter of the textbook.

6. Proceed to the chapter review if your performance rate was 80% or higher, otherwise, return to the chapter for further study.

1.	a	5.	a	9.	a
2.	b	6.	a	10.	a
3.	a	7.	b	11.	b
4.	b	8.	a	12.	a

CHAPTER REVIEW ANSWER KEY

Directions:

1. Correct your Chapter Review Answer Sheet with the answers below by placing a slash (Example: ~~8~~) through the incorrect question number with a pen or pencil of a contrasting color.

2. Record the correct answer to the right of your answer on your answer sheet.

3. Record the total correct on the Initial Performance Grid in section four of this review manual.

4. Calculate your performance rate and also record on the grid.

5. Promptly locate the correct answer for each question missed in the chapter of the textbook.

6. Proceed to the next assigned chapter in your study.

1.	c(10x100)/(51-2)	6.	percentage	11.	median
2.	c(11x100)/(55-2)	7.	b	12.	reliability
3.	a	8.	c	13.	e
4.	mean	9.	b	14.	a
5.	c	10.	a	15.	g

16. b

17. h

18. c

19. f

20. range

21. d

22. b(1,2,4,7,8,11,22)

23. c (22-1)=21

24. d

25. standard deviation or S

26. a

27. c(2226x1000)/110,000

28. d . 02x360=7.2 degrees

29. b(7600x100)/(300x30)

30. d(18x13)+(10x7)+(18x4)/
18+10+18=376/46

31. continuous data or continuous interval data

32. 16.5% (25/152)

33. discrete data

34. Hospital D

35. Hospital C

36. Hospital C

37. ordinal data, ranked data or ranked ordinal data

38. a

39. nominal

40. Medicare

41. 11.8 days
(20+10+7+14+8)/5

42. 15 days
(8,10,15,18,22)

43. population data

44. 195

45. A

46. c

47. a

48. d

QUALITY ASSESSMENT AND IMPROVEMENT

10

PRETEST REVIEW

Directions:

1.   Tear out a Pretest Review Answer Sheet from the back of this review manual.

2.   Read each question carefully before selecting an answer.

3.   Write the correct or best answer on the answer sheet.

4.   Answer all the question,, since there is no penalty for this pretest review.

5.   Check your answers with the answer key located near the end of this chapter.

1.   Five years is the contract period for each PRO *Scope of Work*.

   a.   True
   b.   False

2.   The National Practitioner Data Bank maintains data on the actions of state licensing boards.

   a.   True
   b.   False

3.   The Office of Fiscal and Budgetary Management has jurisdiction over peer review organizations.

   a.   True
   b.   False

4.   Medical record review by the medical staff of the patient care documentation practices of staff physicians is required by the JCAHO to be an on-going process.

   a.   True
   b.   False

5.   Processing reimbursement claims for inpatient services provided to Medicare beneficiaries is the function of the fiscal intermediary.

   a.   True
   b.   False

6.   Report of a potentially compensable event is to risk management as a patient's discharge plan is to utilization management.

   a.   True
   b.   False

7.   Medical staff credentialing is a general function of the medical records committee.

   a.   True
   b.   False

8.   Outlier data points are associated with DRG reimbursement.

   a.   True
   b.   False

9. The *Conditions of Participation* detail regulations governing provider services to Medicare and Medicaid patients.

   a. True
   b. False

10. Every state, by law, protects information generated under peer review processes.

    a. True
    b. False

11. Utilization review is mandated by the federal government and for the accreditation of health care facilities.

    a. True
    b. False

12. The UB-92 captures billing information for fiscal intermediaries.

    a. True
    b. False

CHAPTER REVIEW

Directions:

1.   Tear out a Chapter Review Answer Sheet from the back of this review manual.

2.   Read each question carefully before selecting an answer.

3.   Write the correct or best answer on the answer sheet.

4.   Answer all the questions since there is no penalty in this chapter review.

5.   Check your answers with the answer key located at the end of this chapter review.

1.   _____ is the evaluation of an individual's professional performance by another (or others) of equal professional standing.

2.   The Donabedian Model of Structure, Process and Outcome is conceptualized around three domains which include:

   a.   amenities
   b.   interpersonal
   c.   technological
   d.   both b and c

3.   Which of the following performance evaluation measures examines interaction between patients and providers?

   a.   outcome
   b.   process
   c.   structure
   d.   none of the above

4.   A quality indicator is an objective, quantifiable measurement that targets events, or patterns of events, suggestive of a problematic process or behavior.

   a.   True
   b.   False

5.   A sentinel event is a frequently occurring undesirable outcome warranting further investigation.

   a.   True
   b.   False

6.   When a criterion accurately measures the intended outcome of care and discriminates correctly between the presence and absence of the outcome, it is said to be:

   a.   reliable
   b.   valid
   c.   both reliable and valid
   d.   statistically significant

7.   Intermediate positive pressure breathing (IPPB) is an example of a patient care process that can be evaluated by the utilization review program.

   a.   True
   b.   False

8.   Quality assurance presupposes that a desirable standard of quality in health care cannot be measured as delivered.

   a.   True
   b.   False

9.   Hospitals participating in the Medicare program would find directives regarding required quality assurance activities for Medicare published in all of the following *except:*

   a.   *Accreditation Manual for Health Care Organizations*
   b.   *Conditions of Participation*
   c.   *Federal Register*
   d.   *PRO Scope of Work*

10. The JCAHO mandates a particular methodology for assuring quality of care, such as the IS/SI criteria.

    a. True
    b. False

11. Occurrence screening is a function of utilization review.

    a. True
    b. False

12. Targeted processes and outcomes mandated for quality review by the JCAHO include:

    a. high risk processes
    b. high volume processes
    c. problem prone processes
    d. all of the above

13. Patient care costs associated with "re-work" are generally unrecoverable.

    a. True
    b. False

14. A _____ is an example of "re-work" in the process of delivering health care.

15. Which of the following is *not* associated with clinical review activities required by the JCAHO?

    a. utilization review
    b. medication usage review
    c. medical record review
    d. blood usage review

16. Both an adverse drug reaction and an anesthesia mortality are sentinel events that are subject to intensive quality review.

    a. True
    b. False

17. Medical and nursing staff are required by the JCAHO to participate in:

    a. review of surgical and invasive procedures
    b. medical record review
    c. both a and b
    d. none of the above

18. Medical staff malpractice claims history data and risk profiles are used to establish premium prices for liability insurance coverage.

    a. True
    b. False

19. The principal objective of a Risk Management program is the efficient management of claims against the health care facility.

    a. True
    b. False

20. Credentialing is the process of determining the clinical privileges of physicians on the medical staff.

    a. True
    b. False

21. The ultimate authority for making appointments and granting physician privileges is vested in the:

    a. credentialing committee
    b. executive committee
    c. governing body
    d. chief executive officer

22. The MSO is a self-governing entity.

    a. True
    b. False

23. Physician profiles must be forwarded to the NPDB once annually.

    a. True
    b. False

24. Which category of medical staff membership does *not* include admitting privileges?

    a. active
    b. associate
    c. courtesy
    d. consulting

25. The jurisdiction for medical examination and licensing is vested in the:

    a. State Board of Medical Examiners
    b. National Board of Medical Examiners
    c. executive committee of the medical staff
    d. all of the above

26. MSO bylaws must be approved by the governing board.

    a. True
    b. False

27. The governing body serves as the formal communication link between the executive committee and the medical staff regarding appointments and re/appointments to the staff, especially in smaller facilities having no Joint Conference Committee.

    a. True
    b. False

Most hospitals use generic screening criteria of different types to monitor the quality of care and identify problems. Commonly used criteria are listed below. Match the criteria in the left column with the correct type of criteria in the right column using the abbreviations supplied.

_____ 28. uncontrolled active bleeding at present time

_____ 29. diet tolerated for 24 hours without nausea or vomiting

_____ 30. IV or IM analgesics 3 or more times daily

_____ 31. nosocomial infection

_____ 32. stable hemoglobin/hematocrit

_____ 33. implantation of radioactive material in head, neck, or reproductive organ

_____ 34 sudden onset of functional impairment evidenced by unconsciousness

_____ 35. voiding or draining urine (at least 800cc) for last 24 hours

_____ 36. patient fall resulting in injury

_____ 37. return to ICU within 24 hours of transfer to nursing unit

IS - Intensity of Service Criteria

SI - Severity of Illness Criteria

OS - Occurrence Screening Criteria

DI - Discharge Indicators

Mr. Rocky States was admitted for a BKA of his right leg. Subsequent to surgery he discovered his left leg had been amputated. The hospital Risk Management program is managing the case in cooperation with other hospital services.

38.   Referring to the event above, Mr. States' situation would be termed a(an) _____ by risk management.

39.   Referring to the event above, the situation may be referred to as a _____ because the hospital may be responsible for a financial outlay due to liability or settlement.

40.   Referring to the event above, would the situation necessitate the filing of an incident report?

41.   When incident reports are completed, they are filed in the patient's medical record, with administration and given to the hospital's legal counsel.

   a.   True
   b.   False

42.   The major thrust of the 1989 Omnibus Budget Reconciliation Act was to:

   a.   evaluate unproven processes and techniques
   b.   act as a patient advocacy center for health care consumers
   c.   review claims against providers
   d.   develop clinical practice guidelines

43.   Which is *not* associated with the D*A*T model?

   a.   attitudes
   b.   data
   c.   algorithms
   d.   tools

44.   "Outlier cases" are those cases for which reimbursement for inpatient services is sought beyond the DRG rate and are applicable only to federally-funded patients.

   a.   True
   b.   False

45.   The principal functions of a utilization management program are:

   a.   discharge planning
   b.   concurrent review
   c.   outlier review
   d.   all of the above

46.   IS/SI criteria are applied during:

   a.   concurrent review
   b.   occurrence screening
   c.   retrospective review
   d.   discharge planning

47.   Peer review is required in the criteria setting and problem analysis steps in the QA process.

   a.   True
   b.   False

48.   Which of the following would be of principal interest in the medical staff recredentialing process?

   a.   cost of care compared with DRG reimbursement by physician
   b.   APO's by physician
   c.   outliers by admission
   d.   PRO admission denials by physician

PRETEST REVIEW ANSWER KEY

Directions:

1. Correct your Pretest Review Answer Sheet with the answers below by placing a slash (Example: 8̸) through the incorrect question number with a pen or pencil of a contrasting color.

2. Record the correct answer to the right of your answer on your answer sheet.

3. Record the total correct on the Initial Performance Grid in section four of this review manual.

4. Calculate your performance rate and also record on the grid.

5. Promptly locate the correct answer for each question missed in the chapter of the textbook.

6. Proceed to the chapter review if your performance rate was 80% or higher, otherwise, return to the chapter for further study.

1.	b	5.	a	9.	b
2.	a	6.	a	10.	a
3.	b	7.	b	11.	b
4.	b	8.	a	12.	a

CHAPTER REVIEW ANSWER KEY

Directions:

1. Correct your Chapter Review-Answer Sheet with the answers below by placing a slash (Example: 6̸) through the incorrect question number with a pen or pencil of a contrasting color.

2. Record the correct answer to the right of your answer on your answer sheet.

3. Record the total correct on the Initial Performance Grid in section four of this review manual.

4. Calculate your performance rate and also record on the grid.

5. Promptly locate the correct answer for each question missed in the chapter of the textbook.

6. Proceed to the next assigned chapter in your study.

1.	peer review	6.	b	11.	b
2.	d	7.	b	12.	d
3.	b	8.	b	13.	a
4.	a	9.	a	14.	repeated lab or x-ray; readmission due to complication of care; readmission resulting from premature discharge; others
5.	b	10.	b		

15.	a	28.	SI	39.	PCE
16.	a	29.	DI	40.	Yes
17.	c	30.	IS	41.	b
18.	a	31.	OS	42.	a
19.	b	32.	DI	43.	c
20.	a	33.	IS	44.	b
21.	c	34.	SI	45.	d
22.	a	35.	DI	46.	a
23.	b	36.	OS	47.	b
24.	d	37.	OS	48.	b
25.	a	38.	adverse patient occurrence (APO) or potential compensable event (PCE)		
26.	a				
27.	b				

HEALTH LAW CONCEPTS AND PRACTICES

11

PRETEST REVIEW

Directions:

1.   Tear out a Pretest Review Answer Sheet from the back of this review manual.

2.   Read each question carefully before selecting an answer.

3.   Write the correct or best answer on the answer sheet.

4.   Answer all the questions, since there is no penalty for this pretest review.

5.   Check your answers with the answer key located near the end of this chapter.

1.   Medicare-certified alcohol and drug abuse facilities must comply with *Regulations on Confidentiality of Alcohol and Drug Abuse Patient Records.*

   a.   True
   b.   False

2.   The right of privacy was granted by the U.S. Supreme Court in the Griswold v. Connecticut decision.

   a.   True
   b.   False

3.   In a *tort* action, one party alleges that another party's wrongful conduct has caused him some harm.

   a.   True
   b.   False

4.   In a *contract* action, one party alleges that an agreement existed between himself and another party, and that the other party has breached (broken) that agreement.

   a.   True
   b.   False

5.   A claim against a health care facility for breach of confidentiality could be both a *tort* and a *contract* action.

   a.   True
   b.   False

6.   The right of privacy is expressly guaranteed by the U.S.Constitution.

   a.   True
   b.   False

7. The *plaintiff* is the party who initiates a lawsuit.

   a. True
   b. False

8. The concept of *respondeat superior* refers to holding the employer, supervisor or organization responsible for the actions or inactions of its employees or agents.

   a. True
   b. False

9. Defamation is an example of an intentional tort.

   a. True
   b. False

10. Injecting a patient with medicine against his wishes is an example of fraud.

    a. True
    b. False

11. The length of time health information must be maintained in some form is often dictated by record retention laws and regulations.

    a. True
    b. False

12. A health information professional can *not* be held liable for accidental destruction or loss of a patient's health information.

    a. True
    b. False

CHAPTER REVIEW

Directions:

1. Tear out a Chapter Review —Answer Sheet from the back of this review manual.

2. Read each question carefully before selecting an answer.

3. Write the correct or best answer on the answer sheet.

4. Answer all the questions since there is no penalty in this chapter review.

5. Check your answers with the answer key located at the end of this chapter review.

1. The U.S. Bill of Rights is a source of _____ law.

2. Rules and regulations of administrative agencies such as the DSHS are a source of law.

   a. True
   b. False

3. Invasion of privacy is a tort.

   a. True
   b. False

4. If the surgeons on the medical staff seek to remove a surgeon's staff privileges so that there will be less competition for patients, a claim for respondeat superior can be alleged.

   a. True
   b. False

5. Res ipsa loquitur shifts the burden of proof to the defendant.

   a. True
   b. False

6. The Patient Self-Determination Act legalized assisted suicide, for example.

   a. True
   b. False

7. Living wills are advance directives that are to be maintained with the patient's health information according to the U.S. Bill of Rights.

   a. True
   b. False

8. The admissibility of health information varies with states.

   a. True
   b. False

9. Patient access to their own health information in alcohol and drug abuse treatment facilities is determined by federal law.

   a. True
   b. False

10. In which situation would an informed consent not likely be required providing the circumstances are clearly documented in the patient record?

    a. life-threatening situation
    b. situation of therapeutic privilege
    c. situation in which there is insufficient time before needed treatment
    d. all of the above

Match the terms in the left column with the correct descriptors in the right column. Not all descriptors may have an answer.

_____ 11. interrogatory

_____ 12. discovery

_____ 13. deposition

_____ 14. due process

_____ 15. complaint

_____ 16. contract

_____ 17. arbitration

_____ 18. burden of proof

_____ 19. evidence

_____ 20. pleadings

a. legal document allowing an individual to make decisions regarding their health

b. affidavit of defense is an example

c. deposition is an example

d. written questions under oath

e. a process of resolving disputes outside of court

f. documentation made while care is being provided

g. an enforceable agreement

h. information legally presented at trial

i. the plaintiff's claim that commences a legal action

j. obligation of a party to prove a contention

k. safeguards built into procedures so that individual's rights are protected fairly

l. oral testimony sworn out of court

						NURSES NOTES
					Date: _8/18/8x_	
Time	B. P.	Temp.	Pulse	Resp.	Treatments-Procedures Special Medication P.R.N. Medication	Remarks
1900	150/70		error 96 ~~96~~	24		Sleeping-arowses easily. Oriented to name only. Other neuro assessment unchanged. ————— Nryolds
~~1930~~	142/88		104	24	error 8/18/8x 2000 WBJ	Oriented to name and place. Vest restraint applied.
2000	132/84	99.4	96	24	error 8/18/8x 2000 WBJ	Physical assessment unchanged
2030	130/80		94	24		Earlier assessments un- changed.
2100	134/82		96	24		error 35 W
2200	136/84		104	24	error 8/18/8x	Arowses easily. Side rails up.

21. Referring to the information in the illustration above, which error notation is legally acceptable?

a. the 1900 hour notation
b. the 1930 hour notation
c. the 2000 hour notation
d. the 2200 hour notation

22. A court order requiring someone to come before the court and testify is called a _____.

23. Decisions about who has access to a patient's health information must be made by the patient alone.

    a. True
    b. False

24. Physicians should have free access to a person's health information.

    a. True
    b. False

25. All claims made against health care facilities and health care providers are resolved by the courts.

    a. True
    b. False

26. In deciding cases, courts usually adhere to the principle of *stare decisis*.

    a. True
    b. False

27. The doctrine of charitable immunity for health care organizations has been abolished.

    a. True
    b. False

28. The federal court system is made up of four levels: District Courts, Trial Courts, Courts of Appeals, and the Supreme Court.

    a. True
    b. False

29. Minors who are married, living away from home, responsible for their own support, and who the law recognizes as being able to make their own decisions and agreements are generally called _____.

30. A _____ is a court order requiring someone to come before the court with certain records or documents.

31. If, upon receipt of the court order described in question #30, the HIM professional felt that the order was defective in some way, and the facility wished to contest the validity of that order, what sort of motion would be filed by the facility's legal counsel?

32, 33. In setting facility policies for patient access to their health information, name the two *most* important sources of law that the HIM professional should consult.

34. Record retention schedules should be developed for:

    a. patient records and original xrays
    b. peer review records and minutes
    c. medical staff credential files
    d. a and b only
    e. all of the above

35. In developing a record retention schedule, HIM professionals should consider:

    a. the needs and preferences of the professional staff
    b. the statute of limitations
    c. any state or federal retention statutes or regulations
    d. b and c only
    e. all of the above

36. Mr. Rocky States was admitted to a community hospital for a gallbladder removal. Which information about him is considered confidential?

    a. the patient's health history
    b. the patient's date of birth
    c. the patient's address upon admission
    d. none of the above
    e. all of the above

37. Which of the following is ordinarily found in an inpatient health record?

    a. incident or occurrence report
    b. results of quality reviews done on that case
    c. the problem list
    d. none of the above
    e. all of the above

38. What do federal regulations on the confidentiality of alcohol and drug abuse records apply to?

    a. all health care facilities
    b. identified units providing alcohol or drug abuse diagnosis, treatment, or referrals
    c. medical personnel whose primary function is providing alcohol/drug abuse diagnosis, treatment, or referrals
    d. b and c
    e. none of the above

39. Properly executed authorizations to release alcohol-related treatment information need *not* include:

    a. the name or the program or person permitted to make the disclosure
    b. the party to whom disclosure must be made
    c. the purpose of the disclosure
    d. a description of the information to be disclosed
    e. advance payment for the disclosure

40. Which of the following is an *internal* user of health information:

    a. the facility's quality review committee members
    b. the facility's medical director
    c. the patient
    d. a and b
    e. a, b and c

41. Which of the following parties has ownership interest in a living patient's medical record and the information within it?

    a. the patient's family
    b. the patient
    c. the health care facility
    d. a and b
    e. b and c

42. Which of the following uses of the medical record are typically "impersonal" and do *not* require patient authorization?

    a. use by the facility's quality management program
    b. use by the patient's employer in connection with payment of the bill
    c. use in court to disprove paternity
    d. both a and b

43. When should students and residents in health care professional training programs be permitted access to patient health records?

    a. when the patient authorizes access
    b. when the student or resident provides supervisor authorization
    c. when the student or resident provides facility identification
    d. when the conditions in either a or b are met
    e. under none of these circumstances

44. Which of the following could be categorized as an *administrative* use of the medical record for which authorization by the patient is generally *not* required:

    a. investigation of a patient complaint by the manager of the department involved
    b. review of documentation by the facility's professional liability insurer
    c. review of the record by the patient's attorney
    d. a and b
    e. all of the above

45. Under what circumstance should patients be notified that their health information will be made available to their health insurer?

    a. only when that information is extra-sensitive, e.g., HIV-related tests or treatment, or substance abuse cases
    b. only when that patient is not the person who signed the contract for health insurance
    c. under all circumstances where the health insurer is the payer
    d. under no circumstances

46. Which of the following is *not* part of the minimum recommended content for patient authorization for release of information:

    a. a notice to discuss the release with the attending physician before signing
    b. name of the party to receive the information
    c. signature of the patient (or legal representative)
    d. the date, event, or condition upon which the authorization will expire (unless revoked earlier)
    e. none of the above

47. Confidential health information may be released to law enforcement officers under what circumstances?

   a. when the patient authorizes it
   b. in response to a valid subpoena or court order
   c. either a or b
   d. neither a nor b

48. A 10-year-old child is treated in the emergency room for a broken arm. In cases of divorce and legal separation, consents for treatment and authorizations for release of information about this minor child are ordinarily granted by:

   a. either parent
   b. the parent who arrives at the emergency room first
   c. the parent with legal custody of the child
   d. a or c, depending on the state

PRETEST REVIEW ANSWER KEY

Directions:

1. Correct your Pretest Review Answer Sheet with the answers below by placing a slash (Example:̸8) through the incorrect question number with a pen or pencil of a contrasting color.

2. Record the correct answer to the right of your answer on your answer sheet.

3. Record the total correct on the Initial Performance Grid in section four of this review manual.

4. Calculate your performance rate and also record on the grid.

5. Promptly locate the correct answer for each question missed in the chapter of the textbook.

6. Proceed to the chapter review if your performance rate was 80% or higher, otherwise, return to the chapter for further study.

Answers to Pretest Review

1.	a	5.	a	9.	a
2.	b	6.	b	10.	b
3.	a	7.	a	11.	a
4.	a	8.	a	12.	b

CHAPTER REVIEW ANSWER KEY

Directions:

1. Correct your Chapter Review Answer Sheet with the answers below by placing a slash (Example:̸8) through the incorrect question number with a pen or pencil of a contrasting color.

2. Record the correct answer to the right of your answer on your answer sheet.

3. Record the total correct on the Initial Performance Grid in section four of this review manual.

4. Calculate your performance rate and also record on the grid.

5. Promptly locate the correct answer for each question missed in the chapter of the textbook.

6. Proceed to the next assigned chapter in your study.

Answers to Pretest Review

1.	constitutional	6.	b	11.	d
2.	a	7.	b	12.	c
3.	a	8.	a	13.	l
4.	b	9.	a	14.	k
5.	a	10.	d	15.	i

16.	g	28.	b	36.	a
17.	e	29.	emancipated	37.	c
18.	j	30.	subpoena duces tecum	38.	d
19.	h			39.	e
20.	b or i	31.	motion to quash	40.	d
21.	b			41.	e
22.	subpoena	32.	state statutes, rules & regulations	42.	a
23.	b			43.	d
24.	b	33.	federal laws, rules & regulation	44.	d
25.	b			45.	c
26.	a	34.	e	46.	a
27.	a	35.	e	47.	c
				48.	d

PRINCIPLES OF MANAGEMENT 12

PRETEST REVIEW

Directions:

1. Tear out a Pretest Review-Answer Sheet from the back of this review manual.

2. Read each question carefully before selecting an answer.

3. Write the correct or best answer on the answer sheet.

4. Answer all the questions, since there is no penalty for this pretest review.

5. Check your answers with the answer key located near the end of this chapter.

1. Power is a function of a person's position in an organization.

    a. True
    b. False

2. Behavioral decision theory focuses on the decision maker while normative theory focuses on the process.

    a. True
    b. False

3. Planning involves carefully correcting deviations of actual performance from desired performance.

    a. True
    b. False

4. During the stage setting and preparation phase of planning, the organizational mission should be clearly established.

    a. True
    b. False

5. Long-range plans should logically develop from shorter-range plans.

    a. True
    b. False

6. A budget is an intermediate-range plan.

    a. True
    b. False

7. The formal hierarchy in an organization is called the unified command.

    a. True
    b. False

8. Authority is a person's right to require or prohibit certain actions.

    a. True
    b. False

9. Controlling, like planning and organizing, can be accurately thought of as a process involving several steps.

    a. True
    b. False

10. The difference between the planned desired performance and actual performance is the variance.

    a. True
    b. False

11. Span of control states that organizations benefit most when employees use their natural endowments to do what they do best.

    a. True
    b. False

12. Situational management concepts are an important aspect of the contingency theory of management.

    a. True
    b. False

CHAPTER REVIEW

Directions:

1. Tear out a Chapter Review Answer Sheet from the back of this review manual.

2. Read each question carefully before selecting an answer.

3. Write the correct or best answer on the answer sheet.

4. Answer all the questions since there is no penalty in this chapter review.

5. Check your answers with the answer key located at the end of this Chapter Review.

The Control Process

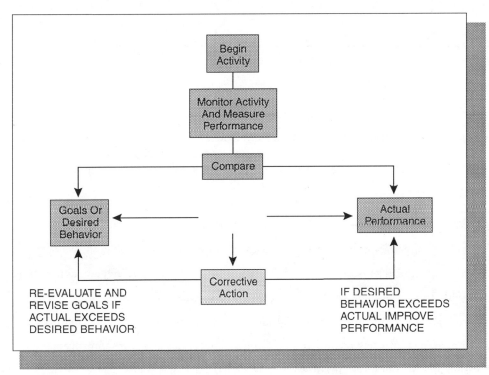

1. Organizations are influenced by how well different groups work together, such as in the _____ system.

2. When leaders make decisions after considering the views of others, a _____ style of leadership is demonstrated.

3. The more decisions are forced to lower levels in the organization, the more _____ it is said to be.

4. Referring to the illustration above, the discrepancy between the desired performance and actual performance is termed _____ and must be measured in this process.

Match the terms in the left column with the correct descriptor in the right column.

_____ 5. forecast	a. self-correcting is an example
_____ 6. job description	b. the identification of accomplishments that are judged to be essential
_____ 7. contingency plan	c. clarifies roles and defines performance standards
_____ 8. performance appraisal	d. measuring a person on the basis of pre-established goals and job-relevant criteria
_____ 9. management by objectives	e. operational and budgetary actions essential for the accomplishment of goals
_____ 10. tactical plan	f. a plan which allows for conditions to vary
_____ 11. strategic plan	g. a result of an analysis of what the organization is presently
_____ 12. feedback control	h. positioning the organization's future in its environmental context
_____ 13. critical success factor	i. the result of determining how likely an alternative is relative to other possible directions
_____ 14. mission	j. participative goal setting and objective evaluation

---

Job Title: Systems Programmer/Technical Support

Classification: Exempt Salaried

Description of Responsibility: Accountable for implementation, maintenance, and evaluation of systems software, telecommunications software and support, and coordination of operations. Accountable for all phases of support of data processing systems functions

Typical Tasks:

1. Develop, plan, implement, and maintain network and data base systems.

2. Evaluate software and hardware changes to enhance and maintain high levels of system performance.

3. Provide technical assistance in areas of problem identification, debugging, and trouble shooting.

4. Provide technical interface among hardware and software vendors, in-house operators, and users.

5. Insure adequate documentation and training on new system software installations.

6. Generate new projects relating to developing technologies and work improvements.

7. Install and maintain system software, utilities, language processors, access methods, and teleprocessing support.

8. Develop, monitor, maintain, and report on system performance measures.

Reporting Relationship: Reports to Associate Administrator and Systems and Programming Manager. Coordinative relationship with Projects Manager.

Qualifications: B. S. degreee in mathematics, computer science, physical sciences, statistics, or accounting. Five years experience in technical data processing and knowledge of data base management, operating system software, data communications, and networking techniques.

---

15. Referring to the information in the illustration on page 126, what is the name for this management tool?

16. Referring to the information in the illustration on page 126, to whom is this employee accountable?

17. Referring to the information in the illustration on page 126, which of the six elements will be used in a performance appraisal?

> The Office of Internal Audit provides consultative and educational services in the identification, evaluation, and control of administrative, operational, financial, informational, compliance, and technological risks. We provide these services to distinct administrative units for the benefit of the Audit Committee of the Board of Directors in an objective, ethical, discreet, and professional manner.

18. Referring to the information in the illustration immediately above, what name is given to this kind of statement?

19. Name one characteristic of an effective management control.

20. The theory of bureaucracy is most often identified with the Frenchman Henri Fayol.

    a. True
    b. False

21. Frederick Taylor is recognized as the "Father of Scientific Management."

    a. True
    b. False

22. Scientific management is accurately referred to as the functional school of thought.

    a. True
    b. False

23. Situational management emphasizes the importance of basing management actions on universal principles of organization.

    a. True
    b. False

24. The process school of management thought viewed management in terms of the functions performed by managers.

    a. True
    b. False

25. The specialization of labor is a sound economic principle that cannot be applied in excess of its value.

    a. True
    b. False

26. The unit of command principle states that employees should *not* have more than one boss at any given time.

    a. True
    b. False

27. The optimum span of management in a hospital emergency room is two doctors and four nurses.

    a. True
    b. False

28. Power is most accurately viewed as what type of process?

    a. influence
    b. authority
    c. management
    d. decision making
    e. none of the above

29. The delegation of authority, if not done appropri-

29. The delegation of authority, if not done appropriately, increases the chance of violating which principle?

    a. unity of command
    b. span of control
    c. hierarchy
    d. specialization
    e. departmentalization

30. The situational theory of organization displays what type of orientation?

    a. absolute
    b. relative
    c. contention
    d. humanistic
    e. both a and c

31. The theory that seeks to understand the relationship between an organization and its environment is the:

    a. classical theory
    b. acceptance theory
    c. imperative theory
    d. contingency theory
    e. confrontation theory

32. Short-range plans usually cover a planning period of approximately:

    a. one year
    b. two years
    c. five years
    d. five to ten years

33. Which of the following is *not* a reason goals (or objectives) are important to organizations:

    a. goals provide a sense of direction
    b. goals always improve performance
    c. goals make improved efficiency possible because they provide a target
    d. goals provide a standard that make control possible

Feedback And Review

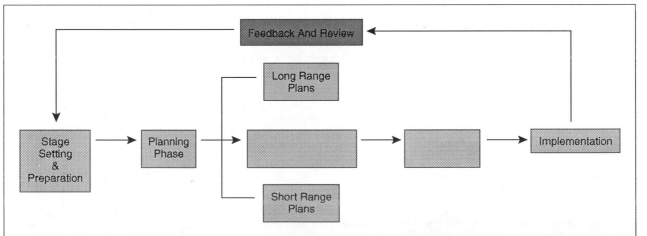

34. Referring to the figure above, what kind of plans should occupy the large rectangle in the center of the figure to complete the planning schema?

35. Referring to the figure above, what kind of plans should occupy the small square, preceeding plan implementation, to complete the planning schema?

36. It is important that managers learn how to delegate authority because it

    a. enables them to shirk their duties
    b. aids in training subordinates
    c. ensures an adequate amount of centralization
    d. makes it clear who has authority

37. Which of the following is *not* a requirement of an effective control?

    a. simplicity
    b. concentration on exceptions
    c. rigidity
    d. cost effectiveness

38. Which of the following functions is *most* important?

    a. planning
    b. organizing
    c. controlling
    d. decision making
    e. none of the above

39. A completely managerial job is more likely to be found at what level in the organization?

    a. top
    b. middle
    c. bottom
    d. none of the above

40. Which of the following is *not* characteristic of the bureaucratic form of organization:

    a. highly specialized
    b. tightly controlled
    c. use of procedures and rules
    d. autonomous

41. Referring to the figure below, the _____ for the Systems Programmer position should be linked to the information in the figure.

Systems Programmer/Technical Support
Critical Success Factors

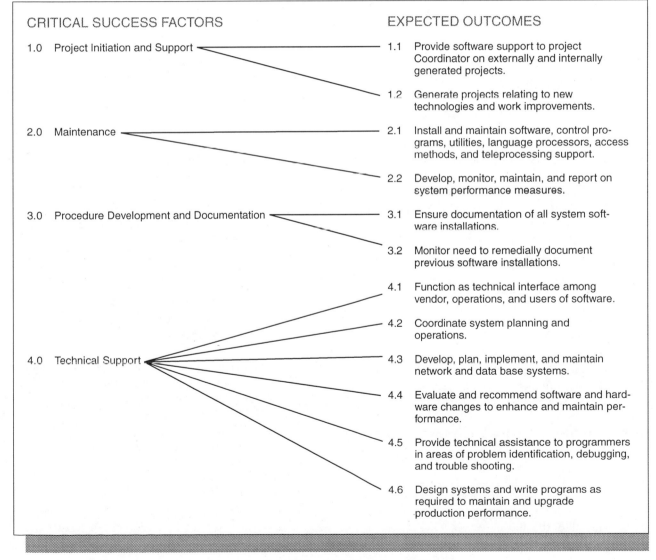

CRITICAL SUCCESS FACTORS

1.0 Project Initiation and Support

2.0 Maintenance

3.0 Procedure Development and Documentation

4.0 Technical Support

EXPECTED OUTCOMES

1.1 Provide software support to project Coordinator on externally and internally generated projects.

1.2 Generate projects relating to new technologies and work improvements.

2.1 Install and maintain software, control programs, utilities, language processors, access methods, and teleprocessing support.

2.2 Develop, monitor, maintain, and report on system performance measures.

3.1 Ensure documentation of all system software installations.

3.2 Monitor need to remedially document previous software installations.

4.1 Function as technical interface among vendor, operations, and users of software.

4.2 Coordinate system planning and operations.

4.3 Develop, plan, implement, and maintain network and data base systems.

4.4 Evaluate and recommend software and hardware changes to enhance and maintain performance.

4.5 Provide technical assistance to programmers in areas of problem identification, debugging, and trouble shooting.

4.6 Design systems and write programs as required to maintain and upgrade production performance.

Office of Internal Audit Critical Success Factors and Objectives/Measures

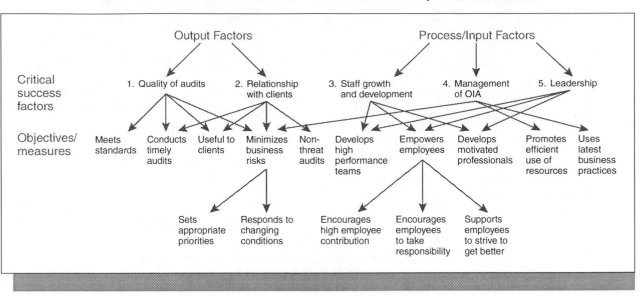

42. Referring to the figure above, the measures illustrated should be linked to the _____ for evaluation of the Internal Auditor.

43. A definition of effective management would require which of the following?

    a. coordination of individual effort
    b. accomplishment of organizational goals
    c. concern for the larger environment
    d. all of the above
    e. a and b only

44. The task of strategic planning in an organization would most likely be completed by:

    a. supervisors
    b. top management
    c. middle managers
    d. consultants
    e. only a and b

45. Variations in the span of management can often be attributed to:

    a. skills of employees
    b. knowledge of manager
    c. working conditions
    d. all of the above
    e. a and c only

46. The number of people a manager can supervise is called the:

    a. limits of authority
    b. authority boundary
    c. power boundary
    d. span of management
    e. b and c

47. The tendency of an organization to make decisions at upper levels is called:

    a. centralization
    b. delegation
    c. decentralization
    d. impersonalization
    e. none of the above

48. When a manager allows another person to exercise a portion of his or her managerial authority, which of the following takes place?

    a. abdication
    b. delegation
    c. leadership
    d. clarification
    e. all of the above

PRETEST REVIEW ANSWER KEY

Directions:

1. Correct your Pretest Review Answer Sheet with the answers below by placing a slash (Example: 8) through the incorrect question number with a pen or pencil of a contrasting color.

2. Record the correct answer to the right of your answer on your answer sheet.

3. Record the total correct on the Initial Performance Grid in section four of this review manual.

4. Calculate your performance rate and also record on the grid.

5. Promptly locate the correct answer for each question missed in the chapter of the textbook.

6. Proceed to the chapter review if your performance rate was 80% or higher, otherwise, return to the chapter for further study.

Answers to Pretest Review

1.	a	5.	b	9.	a
2.	a	6.	b	10.	a
3.	b	7.	b	11.	b
4.	a	8.	a	12.	a

CHAPTER REVIEW ANSWER KEY

Directions:

1. Correct your Chapter Review-Answer Sheet with the answers below by placing a slash (Example: 8) through the incorrect question number with a pen or pencil of a contrasting color.

2. Record the correct answer to the right of your answer on your answer sheet.

3. Record the total correct on the Initial Performance Grid in section four of this review manual.

4. Calculate your performance rate and also record on the grid.

5. Promptly locate the correct answer for each question missed in the chapter of the textbook.

6. Proceed to the next assigned chapter in your study.

Answers to Chapter Review

1.	informal, social or political	6.	c	11.	h
2.	democratic or participative	7.	f	12.	a
3.	decentralized	8.	d	13.	b
4.	varaince	9.	j	14.	g
5.	i	10.	e	15.	job description

16. Associate Administrator & Systems and Programming Manager

17. typical tasks

18. mission statement

19. simple, flexible, economical, or timely

20. b

21. a

22. b

23. b

24. a

25. b

26. a

27. b

28. a

29. a

30. b

31. d

32. a

33. b

34. Intermediate Range Plans

35. Contingency Plans

36. b

37. c

38. e

39. a

40. a

41. job description

42. performance appraisal

43. d

44. b

45. d

46. d

47. a

48. b

HUMAN RELATIONS 13

PRETEST REVIEW

Directions:

1. Tear out a Pretest Review Answer Sheet from the back of this review manual.

2. Read each question carefully before selecting an answer.

3. Write the correct or best answer on the answer sheet.

4. Answer all the questions, since there is no penalty for this pretest review.

5. Check your answers with the answer key located near the end of this chapter.

1. Compromise is the least satisfactory way of dealing with conflict.

   a. True
   b. False

2. Improved communication is associated with worker satisfaction.

   a. True
   b. False

3. Theory X management relies on the "carrot" and "stick" approach to elicit positive worker behavior.

   a. True
   b. False

4. Achilles' heel is a tactic used in team building.

   a. True
   b. False

5. The nominal group process relies on a panel of experts to make predictions

   a. True
   b. False

6. The path/goal model of leadership views the leader as instrumental in facilitating the employee's effort toward desired results.

   a. True
   b. False

7. TQM is a method of monitoring performance over time by charting deviations.

   a. True
   b. False

8. Unresolved conflict forms the foundation of all negotiations.

   a. True
   b. False

9. The decision-making model which applies criteria to the decision process is the Delphi process.

   a.   True
   b.   False

10. "Quality equals zero defects" can be attributed to Crosby's theory.

   a.   True
   b.   False

11. Every negotiations process has common elements such as the need for mediation.

   a.   True
   b.   False

12. A collaborative solution does *not* require follow-up checks.

   a.   True
   b.   False

CHAPTER REVIEW

Directions:

1. Tear out a Chapter Review Answer Sheet from the back of this review manual.

2. Read each question carefully before selecting an answer.

3. Write the correct or best answer on the answer sheet.

4. Answer all the questions since there is no penalty in this chapter review.

5. Check your answers with the answer key located at the end of this chapter review.

1. This decision-making model identifies ideas for priority action:

    a. Delphi process
    b. action-oriented model
    c. Nominal Group Process
    d. brainstorming

2. The process of eliciting the expertise of various constituencies withoutpersonal contact, bias or distortion is accomplished in which decision-making model?

    a. action-oriented model
    b. Delphi process
    c. brainstorming
    d. nominal group process

3. The Theory Y behavior management theory assumes:

    a. people underutilize their natural capacities
    b. people are resistant to applying their energy to the goals of the organization
    c. management must use control methods to ensure productivity
    d. people are motivated by promises and monetary incentives

Match the leadership characteristics in the left column with the correct leadership role in the right column.

_____ 4. The articulation of the organization's mission

_____ 5. The day-to-day exchange between management and the employee

_____ 6. The provision of rewards for effective performance

_____ 7. The process of articulating goals into operating policies, procedures and standards

_____ 8. The creation of a vision for the organization

_____ 9. The provision of resources

_____ 10. The clarification of job requirements

_____ 11. The process of challenging corporate norms and values

_____ 12. The monitoring of employee performance

_____ 13. The use of sanctions for ineffective performance

T1 - Transformational

T2 - Translational

T3 - Transactional

14. The Vroom-Yetton model of leadership employs a decision-making tree emphasizing the process of decision-making.

    a. True
    b. False

15. Conflict resolution can be dealt with by:

    a. avoidance
    b. competition
    c. compromise
    d. all of the above

16. An aggressive problem employee seeks to satisfy personal needs by gunny sacking, moping, fists and tears, and character assassination.

    a. True
    b. False

17. A statistical significance of .10 or .50 is recommended for acceptance levels in hypothesis testing.

    a. True
    b. False

18. A correlation coefficient of +1.0 signifies:

    a. perfect positive correlation between two variables
    b. slight, but insignificant, correlation between two variables
    c. slight, and therefore, a negative relationship between two variables
    d. none of the above

19. This management tool is often used in conjunction with strategic planning by identifying positive and negative effects and the relative effect of each variable on the outcome variable:

    a. affinity diagram
    b. force-field analyses
    c. fishbone diagram
    d. pareto chart

Match the barriers to conflict resolution in the left column with the correct descriptors in the right column. Not all descriptors may have an answer.

_____ 20. Round Robin	a. projecting guilt on the other party
_____ 21. Character Assassination	b. denying a problem exists and avoiding discussion
_____ 22. Hit 'n Run	c. reasserting positions and arguments by both parties resulting in confusion and stalemate
_____ 23. Fists and Tears	d. dwelling on past grievances to strengthen one's position
_____ 24. Gunny Sacking	e. attacking the other person personally rather than discussing the problem
_____ 25. Court Room	f. overwhelming the other party by using an emotional ultimatum
_____ 26. Good Loser	g. hiding one's true feelings for subsequent dumping on the other party
_____ 27. Kitchen Sinking	h. attacking the other personally and then leaving the scene
_____ 28. Silent Treatment	i. bringing in a third party to refute the position of the other
_____ 29. Tempter Tantrum	j. intimidating others through extreme emotion

30. A pareto chart employs a vertical and horizontal axis.

    a. True
    b. False

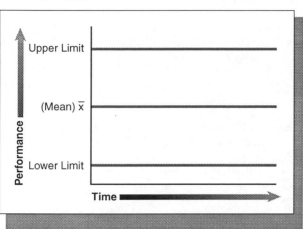

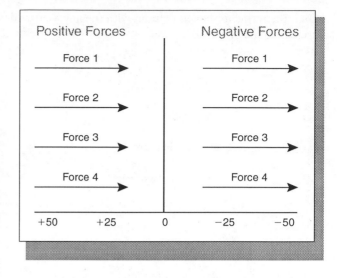

33. Referring to the illustration above, what is the name given to this?

31. Referring to the illustration above, what is the name of this chart?

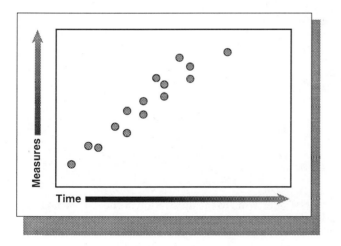

32. Referring to the illustration above, what is the name of this diagram?

Match the terms in the left column with the appropriate descriptor in the right column. Not all descriptors may have an answer.

_____   34. histogram

_____   35. pareto chart

_____   36. affinity diagram

_____   37. force-field analysis

_____   38. run chart

_____   39. control chart

_____   40. fishbone diagram

a.   monitors performance over time by charting deviations of performance

b.   organizes information into homogenous categories for prioritization

c.   graphic representation of sequencial steps in decision-making

d.   multidimensional categorization of qualitative or quantitative data

e.   ordering the relative effect each variable can have on the outcome variable

f.   graphic representation of a frequency distribution

g.   graph representation of data by the use of lines

h.   categorizes occurrences in rank order such as from most to least important

i.   graphic order of probable causes in relation to a defined outcome

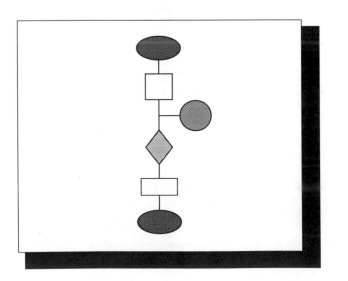

41. Referring to the illustration at the left, what is the name of this diagram?

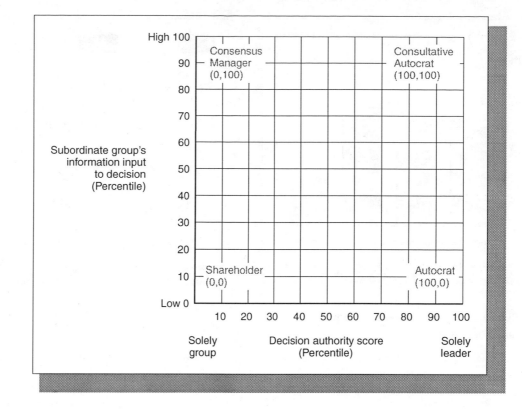

42. Referring to the illustration above, what is the name of this chart?

43. Organizational culture refers to the influence of situational and environmental factors in determining leadership effectiveness.

    a. True
    b. False

44. A Poisson distribution is recommended for use in control charts in health care settings.

    a. True
    b. False

45. Referring to the illustration below, what is the name of this chart?

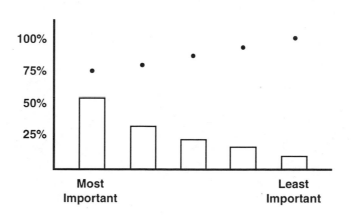

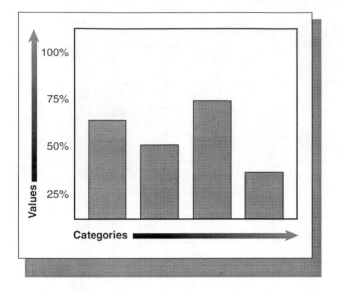

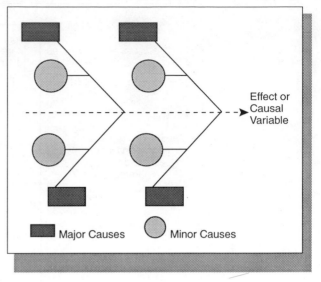

46. Referring to the illustration above, what is the name of this chart?

47. Referring to the illustration above, what is the name of this diagram?

48. The positive and negative relationship of variables is determined by correlation analysis.

    a. True
    b. False

PRETEST REVIEW ANSWER KEY

Directions:

1.   Correct your Pretest Review Answer Sheet with the answers below by placing a slash (Example: 8) through the incorrect question number with a pen or pencil of a contrasting color.

2.   Record the correct answer to the right of your answer on your answer sheet.

3.   Record the total correct on the Initial Performance Grid in section four of this review manual.

4.   Calculate your performance rate and also record on the grid.

5.   Promptly locate the correct answer for each question missed in the chapter of the textbook.

6.   Proceed to the chapter review if your performance rate was 80% or higher, otherwise, return to the chapter for further study.

Answers to Pretest Review

1.	b	5.	b	9.	b
2.	a	6.	a	10.	a
3.	a	7.	b	11.	b
4.	b	8.	a	12.	b

CHAPTER REVIEW ANSWER KEY

Directions:

1.   Correct your Chapter Review Answer Sheet with the answers below by placing a slash (Example: 8) through the incorrect question number with a pen or pencil of a contrasting color.

2.   Record the correct answer to the right of your answer on your answer sheet.

3.   Record the total correct on the Initial Performance Grid in section four of this review manual.

4.   Calculate your performance rate and also record on the grid.

5.   Promptly locate the correct answer for each question missed in the chapter of the textbook.

6.   Proceed to the next assigned chapter in your study.

Answers to Chapter Review

1.	d	6.	T3	11.	T1
2.	b	7.	T2	12.	T3
3.	a	8.	T1	13.	T3
4.	T1	9.	T3	14.	a
5.	T3	10.	T3	15.	d

16.	b	27.	d	38.	g
17.	b	28.	b	39.	a
18.	a	29.	f	40.	i
19.	b	30.	a	41.	affinity
20.	c	31.	control chart	42.	Bonoma-Slevin Leadership Model
21.	e	32.	scatter diagram		
22.	h	33.	force-field analysis	43.	b
23.	j	34.	f	44.	a
24.	g	35.	h	45.	pareto chart
25.	i	36.	b	46.	histogram
26.	a	37.	e	47.	fishbone analysis
				48.	a

HUMAN RESOURCES MANAGEMENT 14

PRETEST REVIEW

Directions:

1. Tear out a Pretest Review Answer Sheet from the back of this review manual.

2. Read each question carefully before selecting an answer.

3. Write the correct or best answer on the answer sheet.

4. Answer all the questions, since there is no penalty for this pretest review.

5. Check your answers with the answer key located near the end of this chapter.

1. The Fair Labor Standards Act makes it illegal to fire an employee for filing a grievance.

    a. True
    b. False

2. Action that follows an infraction is preventive discipline.

    a. True
    b. False

3. The critical incident performance evaluation requires the documentation of good and bad examples of behavior.

    a. True
    b. False

4. The refusal to bargain in good faith with employee representatives constitutes unfair labor activity prohibited by the National Labor Relations Act.

    a. True
    b. False

5. The process of assuring a ready supply of trained help to cover positions when needed is accomplished through job rotation.

    a. True
    b. False

6. A job analysis is a commonly used tool for the development of a Human Resource Plan.

    a. True
    b. False

7. Involuntary termination is the final step in a progressive discipline plan.

    a. True
    b. False

8. A blend of directive and non-directive counseling is called participative employee counseling.

    a. True
    b. False

9. Termination for cause is not grievable.

   a. True
   b. False

10. The elimination of sex-based discrimination in pay practices was mandated by the Fair Labor Standards Act in l938.

    a. True
    b. False

11. A Human Resource Plan prepares the organization for layoffs.

    a. True
    b. False

12. The halo effect is a performance evaluation rater bias.

    a. True
    b. False

CHAPTER REVIEW

Directions:

1. Tear out a Chapter Review Answer Sheet from the back of this review manual.

2. Read each question carefully before selecting an answer.

3. Write the correct or best answer on the answer sheet.

4. Answer all the questions since there is no penalty in this chapter review.

5. Check your answers with the answer key located at the end of this Chapter Review.

1. Which is not a stated goal of health care reform legislation?

    a. increase revenues and profit margins
    b. reduce costs
    c. improve efficiency of services
    d. improve access to services

2. Downsizing of the workforce is generally accomplished through several mechanisms. Which is *not* representative of this process?

    a. reduction in worked hours
    b. voluntary attrition without replacement
    c. involuntary separation
    d. none of the above

3. The process of allowing employees to control their work schedule within parameters established by management is called _____ .

4. Compensation management is regulated by the

    a. JCAHO
    b. National Labor Relations Act
    c. Fair Labor Standards Act
    d. Labor Management Relations Act

5. _____ imposes a duty on employers to provide a safe and healthy workplace.

6. Attracting qualified applicants is an objective of compensation management.

    a. True
    b. False

7. Job sharing occurs when two or more people share a full time position.

    a. True
    b. False

8. Which does not fall under provisions of the Fair Labor Standards Act:

    a. overtime pay
    b. child labor
    c. collective bargaining
    d. record keeping

9. Employees of state and private hospitals are protected by the Age Discrimination in Employment Act.

    a. True
    b. False

10. Which is unrelated to human resource management?

    a. labor relations
    b. staff credentialing
    c. security provisions for staff
    d. employee development

11. Sexual harassment in the workplace is protected by the Fair Labor Standards Act.

    a. True
    b. False

12. The process of fulfilling an organization's mission and goals through human resource management is a functional objective.

    a. True
    b. False

Match the individual elements in the left column with the correct document in the right column using the abbreviations provided.

_____	13.	description of working conditions
_____	14.	summary statement of job
_____	15.	performance standards or criteria
_____	16.	job rank or level
_____	17.	major or essential tasks and responsibilities
_____	18.	position title of the employee
_____	19.	objectives of the job
_____	20.	qualifications for the job
_____	21.	date signed
_____	22.	policies
_____	23.	title of supervisor
_____	24.	signature of supervisor
_____	25.	signature of employee

JA —Job Analysis

JD—Job Description

PA—Performance Appraisal

EM —Employee Manual

ALL—All of the above

26. Aptitude and psychological tests are not performance tests.

   a. True
   b. False

27. New hire screening interviews are generally conducted by the:

   a. hiring supervisor
   b. Human Resource Management Department
   c. management
   d. all of the above

28. Wrongful discharge claims are based on tort law.

   a. True
   b. False

29. Affirmative action programs were promulgated by the ADA.

   a. True
   b. False

30. Attrition refers to voluntary resignation or retirement.

   a. True
   b. False

31. Retaining current competent staff is an objective of compensation management.

   a. True
   b. False

32. Unpaid leave to care for a parent with a serious health condition is protected by federal law.

   a. True
   b. False

Match the statements in the left column with the correct legislation in the right column.

_____ 33. assures reasonable accommodation for impaired persons in the workplace

_____ 34. grants unpaid time off for serious health condition

_____ 35. assures safe and healthful working conditions

_____ 36. sets minimum wage rates

_____ 37. eliminates sex-based discrimination in pay practices

_____ 38. protects against exposure to communicable disease

_____ 39. assures safety of electronic equipment

_____ 40. prohibits interference with formation of a labor organization

_____ 41. prohibits discrimination based on national origin

_____ 42. protects employees and applicants between the ages of 40 and 70

_____ 43. provides equal opportunities in employment for protected groups

_____ 44. prohibits discrimination against qualified individuals with physical or mental impairment

FMLA—Family Medical Leave Act

ADA—Americans with Disabilities Act

OSHA —Occupational Health and Safety Act

FLSA —Fair Labor Standards Act

EPA—Equal Pay Act

NLRA—National Labor Relations Act

CRA—Civil Rights Act

ADEA—Age Discrimination in Employment Act

45. Which must be considered in space planning?

   a. whether more than one person will be using each work station
   b. whether the department/employees will have contact with the public
   c. the amount and type of space needed for each employee
   d. all of the above

46. One type of counseling that may occur in the workplace is _____.

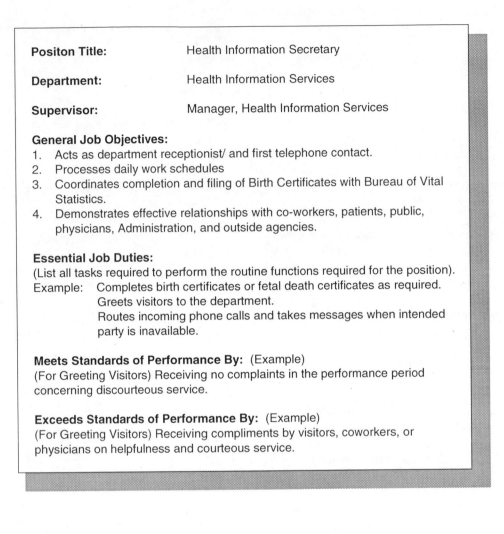

Positon Title: Health Information Secretary

Department: Health Information Services

Supervisor: Manager, Health Information Services

General Job Objectives:
1. Acts as department receptionist/ and first telephone contact.
2. Processes daily work schedules
3. Coordinates completion and filing of Birth Certificates with Bureau of Vital Statistics.
4. Demonstrates effective relationships with co-workers, patients, public, physicians, Administration, and outside agencies.

Essential Job Duties:
(List all tasks required to perform the routine functions required for the position).
Example: Completes birth certificates or fetal death certificates as required.
Greets visitors to the department.
Routes incoming phone calls and takes messages when intended party is inavailable.

Meets Standards of Performance By: (Example)
(For Greeting Visitors) Receiving no complaints in the performance period concerning discourteous service.

Exceeds Standards of Performance By: (Example)
(For Greeting Visitors) Receiving compliments by visitors, coworkers, or physicians on helpfulness and courteous service.

47. Referring to the illustration above, what is the name of this form?

48. Referring to the illustration on the following pages, what is the name of this form?

Name: _____   **Title:** _____

1. Ensure audits are consistent with internal audit standards	Performed Below Expectation	Performed As Expected	Performed Above Expectation

Comments/Recommendations:

_____

_____

_____

2. Ensures audits are timely	Performed Below Expectation	Performed As Expected	Performed Above Expectation

Comments/Recommendations:

_____

_____

_____

3. Ensures audits are useful to clients	Performed Below Expectation	Performed As Expected	Performed Above Expectation

Comments/Recommendations:

_____

_____

_____

4. Sets appropriate audit priorities	Performed Below Expectation	Performed As Expected	Performed Above Expectation

Comments/Recommendations:

_____

_____

_____

5. Responds appropriately to changing conditions in the department and the medical center	Performed Below Expectation	Performed As Expected	Performed Above Expectation

Comments/Recommendations:

_____

_____

_____

6. Interacts with and reports to clients in a consultative manner	Performed Below Expectation	Performed As Expected	Performed Above Expectation

Comments/Recommendations:

7. Nurtures high performing teams	Performed Below Expectation	Performed As Expected	Performed Above Expectation

Comments/Recommendations:

_____

_____

_____

8. Encourages employees to take responsibility for their actions	Performed Below Expectation	Performed As Expected	Performed Above Expectation

Comments/Recommendations:

_____

_____

_____

9. Supports employees to strive to get better at what they do	Performed Below Expectation	Performed As Expected	Performed Above Expectation

Comments/Recommendations:

_____

_____

_____

10. Provides an environment that encourages motivation	Performed Below Expectation	Performed As Expected	Performed Above Expectation

Comments/Recommendations:

_____

_____

_____

11. Utilizes resources efficiently	Performed Below Expectation	Performed As Expected	Performed Above Expectation

Comments/Recommendations:

_____

_____

_____

12. Uses the appropriate business practices	Performed Below Expectation	Performed As Expected	Performed Above Expectation

Comments/Recommendations:

_____

_____

_____

OVERALL RATING	Performed Below Expectation	Performed As Expected	Performed Above Expectation

Comments/Recommendations:

_____

_____

_____

Evaluated by:_____ Title: _____ Date: _____

PRETEST REVIEW ANSWER KEY

Directions:

1. Correct your Pretest Review Answer Sheet with the answers below by placing a slash (Example: 8̸) through the incorrect question number with a pen or pencil of a contrasting color.

2. Record the correct answer to the right of your answer on your answer sheet.

3. Record the total correct on the Initial Performance Grid in section four of this review manual.

4. Calculate your performance rate and also record on the grid.

5. Promptly locate the correct answer for each question missed in the chapter of the textbook.

6. Proceed to the chapter review if your performance rate was 80% or higher, otherwise, return to the chapter for further study.

Answers to Pretest Review

1.	b	5.	a	9.	a
2.	b	6.	b	10.	b
3.	a	7.	a	11.	b
4.	a	8.	a	12.	a

CHAPTER REVIEW ANSWER KEY

Directions:

1. Correct your Chapter Review Answer Sheet with the answers below by placing a slash (Example: 8̸) through the incorrect question number with a pen or pencil of a contrasting color.

2. Record the correct answer to the right of your answer on your answer sheet.

3. Record the total correct on the Initial Performance Grid in section four of this review manual.

4. Calculate your performance rate and also record on the grid.

5. Promptly locate the correct answer for each question missed in the chapter of the textbook.

6. Proceed to the next assigned chapter in your study.

Answers to Chapter Review

1.	a	6.	a	11.	b
2.	d	7.	a	12.	b
3.	flex-time	8.	c	13.	JD
4.	c	9.	a	14.	JD
5.	OSHA	10.	b	15.	PA, JA or JD

16. JD

17. JD or JA

18. JA, JD or PA

19. JA

20. JD

21. PA

22. EM

23. JA or JD

24. PA

25. PA or EM (while the employee manual itself is not signed, the employee must sign a statement that he/ she has received, read and addressed questions about the manual)

26. a

27. a

28. a

29. b

30. a

31. a

32. a

33. ADA

34. FMLA

35. OSHA

36. NLRA

37. EPA

38. OSHA

39. OSHA

40. NLRA

41. CRA

42. ADEA

43. CRA

44. ADA

45. d

46. directive, non-directive or participative

47. job analysis

48. performance evaluation or performance appraisal

FINANCIAL MANAGEMENT

15

PRETEST REVIEW

Directions:

1. Tear out a Pretest Review Answer Sheet from the back of this review manual.

2. Read each question carefully before selecting an answer.

3. Write the correct or best answer on the answer sheet.

4. Answer all the questions, since there is no penalty for this pretest review.

5. Check your answers with the answer key located near the end of this chapter.

1. An organization's equity and liabilities are located on its balance sheet.

   a. True
   b. False

2. The proposed outlay for an automated Master Patient Index would be found in the capital budget.

   a. True
   b. False

3. The management tool that predicts when cash will be received and dispersed is a chart of accounts.

   a. True
   b. False

4. The specific budget that determines sources and uses of cash is called the operating budget.

   a. True
   b. False

5. The proposed outlay for a DRG Encoder would be found in the operating budget.

   a. True
   b. False

6. Estimating gross operating revenues is a major phase in developing the Business Plan.

   a. True
   b. False

7. A profit center is a type of responsibility center where inputs, revenues and expenses are measured.

   a. True
   b. False

8. On April 1, Rocky Mountain Hospital is obligated to pay the final balance of $2,500 for the purchase of new PCs. The amount owed is considered a liability.

   a. True
   b. False

9. FTE expenses are figured in the operating budget.

    a. True
    b. False

10. The accrual accounting method records revenues as they are received.

    a. True
    b. False

11. The denominator for calculating current ratio is *current liabilities*.

    a. True
    b. False

12. The numerator for calculating the operating margin ratio is the *expenses required to supply the revenues*.

    a. True
    b. False

CHAPTER REVIEW

Directions:

1. Tear out a Chapter Review Answer Sheet from the back of this review manual.

2. Read each question carefully before selecting an answer.

3. Write the correct or best answer on the answer sheet.

4. Answer all the questions since there is no penalty in this chapter review.

5. Check your answers with the answer key located at the end of this chapter review.

1. To analyze what has actually been expended compared with that which was budgeted can be determined from the _____ report.

2. The CFO asks you to compare the value of purchasing new high speed photocopying equipment to contracted copying services. What capital expenditure evaluation method would you employ?

3. The CFO is largely responsible for:

   a. managerial finance
   b. managerial accounting
   c. financial accounting
   d. cost accounting

4. The duties of the controller include:

   a. planning investment
   b. securing financing
   c. preparing budgets
   d. recording financial transactions

5. The balance sheet does *not* display:

   a. assets
   b. equity
   c. liabilities
   d. revenues

6. An organization can measure its ability to meet its short and long-term obligations by calculating its:

   a. capitalization ratio
   b. liquidity ratio
   c. both a and b
   d. neither a or b

7. The current ratio can be calculated from the:

   a. chart of accounts
   b. balance sheet
   c. statement of revenues and expenses
   d. variance report

8. Ratio analysis includes:

   a. activity
   b. liquidity
   c. production
   d. all of the above

9. When the current ratio is 3:1:

   a. the payback period is 3 years
   b. the amount of cash and liquid assets needed to meet bills is three times what is needed
   c. the expense required to supply needed revenue will be three times the net revenue
   d. a 3% return on your investment will be realized

10. A health care organization's profit or loss can be determined from the:

    a. fund balance
    b. balance sheet
    c. statement of revenue and expenses
    d. income statement

11. The master budget is a consolidation of the:

    a. statistical, operating, cash and capital budgets
    b. department capital budgets
    c. department operating budgets
    d. department capital and operating budgets

12. When the CFO makes reference to "weighing opportunity costs", he/she is referring to the next best alternative use of investment funds.

    a. True
    b. False

13. Which budgeting approach requires a description of consequences if health care programs or services are terminated or reduced?

    a. rolling
    b. zero-based
    c. flexible
    d. both b and c

14. Rocky Mountain Hospital wants to evaluate how well its resources are being used for the new Sports Medicine Clinic. Which ratio analysis would supply the needed information?

    a. activity ratio
    b. current ratio
    c. capitalization ratio
    d. operating margin ratio

15. Depreciation expense is considered a cash outflow.

    a. True
    b. False

16. Cash outflows and inflows are related to the accounting rate of return.

    a. True
    b. False

17. Capital evaluation methods include:

    a. net present value
    b. payback period
    c. both a and b
    d. neither a or b

18. The double-distribution method of allocation assumes that the allocation of costs cannot be linear.

    a. True
    b. False

19. Which is a patient-revenue generating departments(s) in a fee-for-service health care environment?

    a. physical therapy
    b. laboratory
    c. both a and b
    d. neither a or b

20. Health Information Services and Admitting Services are considered non-patient revenue generating departments.

    a. True
    b. False

21. The process of allocating the costs of non-patient revenue generating departments to patient revenue generating departments can be accomplished by which method?

    a. step-down method
    b. double-distribution method
    c. simultaneous-equations method
    d. all of the above

22. A flexible budget adjusts for the impact of volume changes.

    a. True
    b. False

23. Prospective payment is based on actual charges for delivering services that are fixed in advance.

    a. True
    b. False

24. The statistics budget provides input for the development of the expense budget and the revenue budget.

    a. True
    b. False

Match the terms in the left column with the correct descriptor in the right column. Not all descriptors may have answers.

_____	25. charge master	a. the time frame that must pass before inflow of cash equals or exceeds the outflow
_____	26. gross patient revenue	b. charges for services provided
_____	27. net income	c. the comparison of projects by the discounted value of all cash inflows and outflows
_____	28. net present value	d. money received today is worth more than same amount some period from today
_____	29. net working capital	e. money received less cost of service assuming cost is less than revenue
_____	30. opportunity costs	f. current assets less current liabilities
_____	31. payback period	g. excess of all revenues less all expenses for a period
_____	32. profit	h. excess of all expenses over all revenues for a period
_____	33. revenue	i. amount of revenues expected to be received
_____	34. time value of money	j. master charge list
		k. charges for all patient services not reduced by discounts, allowances, or other adjustments
		l. the amount needed to be deposited today in order to have designated amount at end of period
		m. benefits that would be received from the next best use of the funds

35. One of the financial statements most useful to the Director of Health Information Management is the _____.

36. Which financial statement depicts the financial condition of an organization as of one date in time?

37. Which financial statement depicts the financial activity of an organization for a period of time?

38. Rocky Mountain Health Information Services Department purchased five automobiles for use in delivering records from its centralized location to the twenty clinics it serves in the community. Each of the clinics have an option of hiring its own courier to deliver and retrieve mail sent to the central location or use the Health Information Services delivery vehicle. Each clinic has chosen to use the Health Information Services option. Each car cost $12,000 and has an estimated useful life of three years.

The Accounting Department uses straight line depreciation. The Health Information Services Department anticipates that each car will be used to make 1,500 mail deliveries per year. For each mail delivery there will be a charge of $3.00 that can be applied toward a future purchase of a replacement vehicle. What is the payback period for the cars?

39. _____ is an example of variable costs.

40. _____ is an example of fixed costs.

ROCKY MOUNTAIN HOSPITAL
Balance Sheet
12/31/9X

Assets	199X
Current Assets*	$ 2,438,776
Fixed Assets	5,874,231
Other Assets	558,432
Total Assets	$ 8,871,439

Liabilities and Fund Balances

Current Liabilities	
Accounts and notes payable	$ 345,798
Staffing and payroll-related	841,621
Other short term payables	10,102
Total Current Liabilities	$ 1,197,521
Long Term Liabilities	
Long-term debt	$ 5,950,728
Note payable	2,000,000
Total Long Term Liabilities	$ 7,950,728
Total Liabilities	$ 9,148,249
Fund Balance	$ (276,810)
Total Liabilities and Fund Balance	$ 8,871,439

*Includes $1,438,776 in patient accounts receivable

ROCKY MOUNTAIN HOSPITAL
Income Statement
1/1/9X–12/31/9X

Revenues from Operations	199X
Patient Services	$ 2,855,500
Less Contractual Allowances	24,645
Net Patient Service Revenue	$ 2,830,865
Net Other Revenues	123,744
Total Revenue from Operations	$ 2,954,609

Expenses form Operations	
Salaries and Expenses	$ 1,124,818
Management Salaries and Expenses	305,720
Other Salaries and Expenses	213,412
Supplies and Books	486,257
Utilities	38,110
Depreciation	542,333
Interest and Other	305,124
Total Expenses from Operations	$ 3,015,774

41. Referring to the information in the tables on the previous page, compute the current ratio.

42. Referring to the information in the tables on the previous page, compute the operating margin ratio.

43. Referring to the information in the tables on the previous page, compute the days of revenue in patient accounts receivable.

44. Referring to the information in the tables on the previous page, compute the return on assets.

45. A free-standing ambulatory care center incurs medical record folder costs of $3 per new patient and has a monthly rent payment on its space of $12,000. Which of these is a variable cost?

46. Referring to the information in question #45, which is a fixed cost?

47. What is 'the' accounting equation that is fundamental to financial management?

48. Budgeting is one of the three stages of _____.

PRETEST REVIEW ANSWER KEY

Directions:

1. Correct your Pretest Review Answer Sheet with the answers below by placing a slash (Example: 8) through the incorrect question number with a pen or pencil of a contrasting color.

2. Record the correct answer to the right of your answer on your answer sheet.

3. Record the total correct on the Initial Performance Grid in section four of this review manual.

4. Calculate your performance rate and also record on the grid.

5. Promptly locate the correct answer for each question missed in the chapter of the textbook.

6. Proceed to the chapter review if your performance rate was 80% or higher, otherwise, return to the chapter for further study.

Correct Answers to Pretest Review

1.	a	5.	a	9.	a
2.	a	6.	b	10.	b
3.	b	7.	b	11.	a
4.	b	8.	a	12.	b

CHAPTER REVIEW ANSWER KEY

Directions:

1. Correct your Chapter Review Answer Sheet with the answers below by placing a slash (Example: 8) through the incorrect question number with a pen or pencil of a contrasting color.

2. Record the correct answer to the right of your answer on your answer sheet.

3. Record the total correct on the Initial Performance Grid in section four of this review manual.

4. Calculate your performance rate and also record on the grid.

5. Promptly locate the correct answer for each question missed in the chapter of the textbook.

6. Proceed to the next assigned chapter in your study.

Correct Answers to Chapter Review

1.	variance	6.	b	11.	c
2.	net present value	7.	b	12.	a
3.	a	8.	d	13.	b
4.	c	9.	b	14.	d
5.	d	10.	c	15.	a

16.	b	30.	m	41.	2.04 - $2,438,776/$1,197,521
17.	c	31.	c	42.	(2.07) - ($2,954,609 - $3,015,774) = ($61,165)/$2,954,609
18.	b	32.	e or g		
19.	c	33.	b		
20.	a	34.	a	43.	185.5 days $1,438,776/ ($2,830,865/365) $7,755.79
21.	d	35.	statement of revenues and expenses and balance sheet		
22.	a			44.	(.7%) ($61,165)/$8,871,439
23.	b	36.	balance sheet		
24.	a	37.	statement of revenues and expenses	45.	folders
25.	j			46.	rent
26.	k	38.	2.67 years ($3.00 x 1500) del./yr. = $4,500; $12,000/$4,500	47.	assets = liabilities + owner's equity + revenue − expenses
27.	g				
28.	d	39.	materials or supplies		
29.	f	40.	rent, depreciation, or interest	48.	planning

METHODS FOR ANALYZING AND IMPROVING SYSTEMS

16

PRETEST REVIEW

Directions:

1. Tear out a Pretest Review Answer Sheet from the back of this review manual.

2. Read each question carefully before selecting an answer.

3. Write the correct or best answer on the answer sheet.

4. Answer all the questions, since there is no penalty for this pretest review.

5. Check your answers with the answer key located near the end of this chapter.

1. A major objective of systems analysis and systems design is efficient utilization of resources.

   a. True
   b. False

2. In the input-output cycle of a system, feedback is a process of contrasting what was produced to what should have been produced.

   a. True
   b. False

3. Interpersonal and political relationships make up the formal organization.

   a. True
   b. False

4. A flow process chart shows the flow of work.

   a. True
   b. False

5. A decision grid compares one organization's performance with the performance of another.

   a. True
   b. False

6. Work standards are used to measure actual performance and not to specify expected performance.

   a. True
   b. False

7. A PERT chart is used to give likely completion times for units of work.

   a. True
   b. False

8. The process of making a dramatic change and improvement in performance after re-evaluation is a theory of management called re-engineering.

   a. True
   b. False

9. The consecutive handling of tasks is called serial work division.

    a. True
    b. False

10. The display of the tasks performed by a workgroup and the individual employees in a workgroup is accomplished by a work distribution chart.

    a. True
    b. False

11. Productivity can be measured by dividing inputs by outputs.

    a. True
    b. False

12. Systems design is a component of systems analysis.

    a. True
    b. False

CHAPTER REVIEW

Directions:

1. Tear out a Chapter Review Answer Sheet from the back of this review manual.

2. Read each question carefully before selecting an answer.

3. Write the correct or best answer on the answer sheet.

4. Answer all the questions since there is no penalty in this chapter review.

5. Check your answers with the answer key located at the end of this chapter review.

1. Productivity can be increased by increasing resources and decreasing output.

    a. True
    b. False

2. The informal organization is designed to plan work, assign responsibility, supervise work, and measure results.

    a. True
    b. False

3. Which of the following is *not* characteristic of the formal organization?

    a. illustrates lines of authority
    b. gives the employees a greater understanding of the formal structure
    c. illustrates the everyday interaction between employees
    d. illustrates span of control

4. A well known benefit of the informal organization is that it provides an additional channel of communication.

    a. True
    b. False

5. Which of the following is an advantage of the informal organization?

    a. group discussions can be linked to TQM
    b. can be easily depicted on an organizational chart
    c. Aids in the idetification of overlapping responsibilities
    d. work group can develop cross purposes with the formal organization

6. Which is a major objective for utilizing systems analysis and systems design?

    a. efficient utilization of resources
    b. control operating costs
    c. improve operations
    d. attain major objectives
    e. all of the above

7. Which of the following is an advantage of departmental systems analysis and systems design?

    a. better coordination of functions
    b. elimination of unproductive activities
    c. improvement of operating efficiency
    d all of the above.

8. Systems design is performed to improve an existing system or to create a new system.

    a. True
    b. False

9. Examples of output include labor, energy, and money.

    a. True
    b. False

10. Which phase of systems design is sometimes called transformation?

    a. input
    b. output
    c. processing
    d. feedback

11. Which phase of systems design monitors and compares output with standards of performance?

    a. input
    b. output
    c. processing
    d. feedback

12. Which refers to the use of common sense concepts to eliminate waste of time, energy, material, equipment, and space in the performance of a task?

    a. system analysis
    b. productivity
    c. work simplification
    d. systems design

13. What is the first basic step in work simplification?

14. What is the last basic step in work simplification?

15. An operation flow chart delineates the flow of data through the system.

    a. True
    b. False

16. The purpose of a movement diagram is to depict the flow of work through the physical environment in which the work process is performed.

    a. True
    b. False

17. Which is an analytical tool that provides a means of communication about the logical sequence of a particular operation?

    a. decision table
    b. decision grid
    c. decision tree
    d. decision tool

18. The main objective of BPR is to:

    a. reduce cost
    b. increase revenue
    c. improve quality
    d. reduce risk
    e. all of the above

19. Which is a tool that displays the step-by-step activities in a particular process?

    a. movement diagram
    b. operation flow chart
    c. systems flow chart
    d. process flow chart

20,21
List two characteristics of projects.

22. The definition phase of project planning identifies the:

    a. problem statement
    b. goal
    c. objective
    d. resources
    e. all of the above

23. In project planning, what components should be included in the plan document?

    a. project activities, activity sequence, and project proposal
    b. project activities, time and cost, activity sequences, critical activities, project proposal
    c. activities, time and cost, proposal
    d. project activities, critical activities, proposal

24. Which is the first phase in the implementation process of project management?

    a. problem identification
    b. control
    c. organization
    d. none of the above

25. Which is a scheduling tool that is a system of diagramming steps or component parts of a complex project?

    a. PERT chart
    b. Gantt chart
    c. process flow chart
    d. decision tree

26. Which is a scheduling tool that consists of a horizontal scale divided into units of time and a vertical scale depicting project work elements?

    a. PERT chart
    b. Gantt chart
    c. process flow chart
    d. decision tree

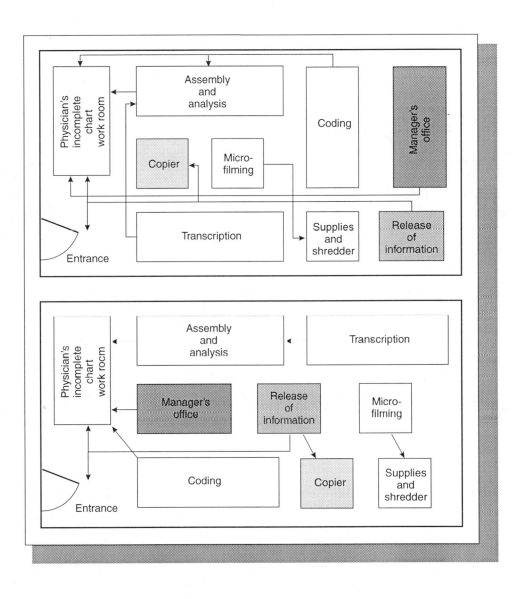

27. Referring to the illustration above, what is the name of this diagram?

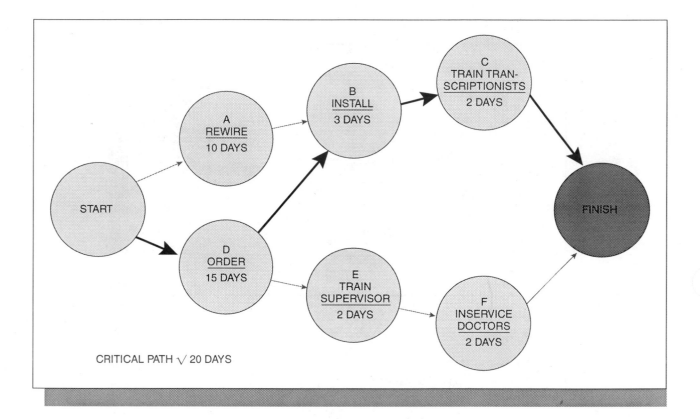

CRITICAL PATH √ 20 DAYS

28. Referring to the illustration immediately above, what is the name of this chart?

29. Referring to the illustration immediately above, how many critical path days would be required to install the new dictation equipment?

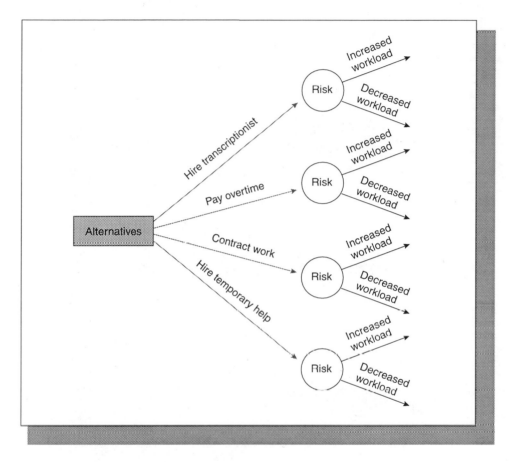

30. Referring to the illustration immediately above, what is the name of this diagram?

31. Referring to the illustration immediately above, would you agree that its purpose is to compare various alternatives in a decision against criteria for making the decision?

    a. Yes
    b. No

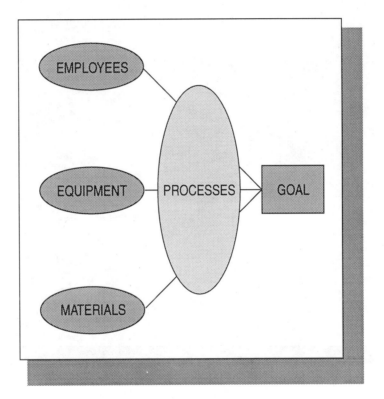

32. Referring to the illustration immediately above, what is the name of this chart?

33. Referring to the illustration immediately above, how many minutes were reduced by the proposed change in release of information delays?

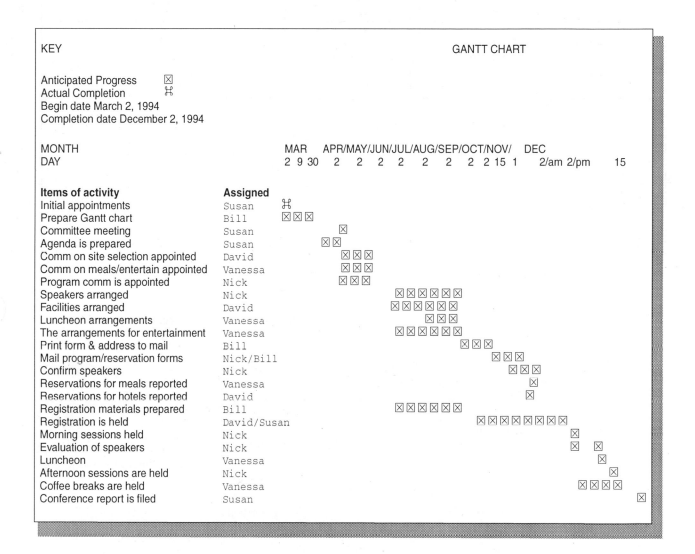

34. Referring to the illustration immediately above, what is the name of this chart?

35. Referring to the illustration immediately above, which activity is expected to take the longest?

36. Referring to the illustration immediately above, which employee is expected to be the busiest in scheduling conferences?

Alternative	Cost	Feasibility	Desirability & Acceptance	Decision
1. Hire new coding supervisor	$28,000 position	Requires recruitment; few qualified applicants; usually new grad	coding staff will resist new graduate	
2. Promote lead coder to coding supervisor	$8,000 Raise ($28,000) $20,000 savings	Places heavy burden on work load	Coding staff may resist	
3. Promote operations supervisor to Assist. Director supervising both operations and coding	$12,000 Raise ($28,000) $16,000 savings	Excellent; supervisor has previous coding experience	Poses minor acceptance problem with coders; very desirable to operations supervisor	

37. Referring to the illustration immediately above, what is the name of this chart?

38. Referring to the information in the illustration above, which alternative should receive first priority?

39. All of the following are methods of work division *except:*

    a. territory
    b. system
    c. function
    d. process

40. Serial, parallel, and unit assembly are:

    a. methods of lower level work division
    b. mid-management planning methods
    c. control processes
    d. systems and subsystems

41. Dividing up work among employees demonstrates which management function?

    a. planning
    b. organizing
    c. directing
    d. controlling

42. The *serial* work distribution method demonstrates _____ handling of the work to be accomplished.

    a. congruent
    b. simultaneous
    c. direct
    d. consecutive

43. The *parallel* work distribution method demonstrates _____ handling of the work to be accomplished.

    a. congruent
    b. simultaneous
    c. direct
    d. consecutive

44. The *unit assembly* method demonstrates _____ handling of the work to be accomplished.

    a. congruent
    b. simultaneous
    c. direct
    d. consecutive

45. Which is a spreadsheet or matrix illustrating the tasks being performed in an organization?

    a. movement diagram
    b. productivity chart
    c. right and left hand chart
    d. work distribution chart

46. Who primarily benefits from an analysis of work distribution charts?

    a. department head
    b. employees whose work is involved
    c. supervisor
    d. director of human resources

47. Which is an advantage of the work distribution chart?

    a. it shows how much time an employee spends on a task
    b. it shows whether work is being evenly distributed
    c. it shows which tasks take the most time to complete
    d. all of the above

48. What is the first step in a productivity improvement program?

    a. establishing a unit of measurement for the work
    b. selecting the area to be improved
    c. analyzing results
    d. developing a measurable productivity objective

PRETEST REVIEW ANSWER KEY

Directions:

1. Correct your Pretest Review Answer Sheet with the answers below by placing a slash (Example:⁄8) through the incorrect question number with a pen or pencil of a contrasting color.

2. Record the correct answer to the right of your answer on your answer sheet.

3. Record the total correct on the Initial Performance Grid in section four of this review manual.

4. Calculate your performance rate and also record on the grid.

5. Promptly locate the correct answer for each question missed in the chapter of the textbook.

6. Proceed to the chapter review if your performance rate was 80% or higher, otherwise, return to the chapter for further study.

Answers to Pretest Review

1.	a	5.	b	9.	a
2.	a	6.	b	10.	a
3.	b	7.	a	11.	b
4.	b	8.	a	12.	b

CHAPTER REVIEW ANSWER KEY

Directions:

1. Correct your Chapter Review Answer Sheet with the answers below by placing a slash (Example:⁄8) through the incorrect question number with a pen or pencil of a contrasting color.

2. Record the correct answer to the right of your answer on your answer sheet.

3. Record the total correct on the Initial Performance Grid in section four of this review manual.

4. Calculate your performance rate and also record on the grid.

5. Promptly locate the correct answer for each question missed in the chapter of the textbook.

6. Proceed to the next assigned chapter in your study.

Answers to Chapter Review

1.	b	6.	e	11.	d
2.	b	7.	d	12.	c
3.	c	8.	a	13.	select an area of work
4.	a	9.	b	14.	apply new or improved method
5.	a	10.	c		

15. b

16. a

17. a

18. e

19. d

20., 21. (any two)
  unique; have one clear goal; product or result-oriented; finite; complex; involve change; employ team approach; use limited resources

22. e

23. b

24. c

25. a

26. b

27. movement diagram

28. PERT chart

29. 19 days

30. decision tree

31. b

32. process flow chart or flow process chart

33. 30 minutes

34. Gantt chart

35. registration

36. Nick

37. decision grid

38. alternative #3

39. b

40. a

41. b

42. d

43. a

44. b

45. d

46. c

47. d

48. b

COMPUTER-BASED PATIENT RECORD
A UNIFYING PRINCIPLE

17

PRETEST REVIEW

Directions:

1. Tear out a Pretest Review Answer Sheet from the back of this review manual.

2. Read each question carefully before selecting an answer.

3. Write the correct or best answer on the answer sheet.

4. Answer all the questions, since there is no penalty for this pretest review.

5. Check your answers with the answer key located near the end of this chapter.

1. Communications and networking applications are components of a comprehensive health information system.

    a. True
    b. False

2. HELP was one of the earliest information systems to replace the patient paper record.

    a. True
    b. False

3. An information warehouse receives data from various transaction systems and combines it with other organization data.

    a. True
    b. False

4. Bedside workstations are a component of a point of care information system.

    a. True
    b. False

5. Momentum was added to the development of computer-based patient records by the recommendations of the IOM Study on this topic.

    a. True
    b. False

6. Terminals employ methods of selecting and entering data by the use of a keyboard and by pointing, clicking and touching input devices.

    a. True
    b. False

7. Most single users of computers use minicomputers.

    a. True
    b. False

8. The operating system is that component of the CPU which is activated by software.

    a. True
    b. False

9. LANs utilize servers to link PCs to mainframes.

   a. True
   b. False

10. Data structures contain one or more databases.

   a. True
   b. False

11. Encoders extract information from databases for analysis and reformating.

   a. True
   b. False

12. Many biomedical devices are used to measure physical changes in the human body and report those findings electronically to the CPR.

   a. True
   b. False

CHAPTER REVIEW

Directions:

1. Tear out a Chapter Review Answer Sheet from the back of this review manual.

2. Read each question carefully before selecting an answer.

3. Write the correct or best answer on the answer sheet.

4. Answer all the questions since there is no penalty in this chapter review.

5. Check your answers with the answer key located at the end of this chapter review.

1. The American National Standards Institute coordinates the activities of voluntary standards-setting systems and organizations.

    a. True
    b. False

2. A printer is an input and an output device.

    a. True
    b. False

3. A disc drive reads software and data files into memory.

    a. True
    b. False

4. Interfaced information systems are characterized by:

    a. a common database shared by all departments
    b. a single data dictionary
    c. both a and b
    d. none of the above

5. The organizational trend is to combine analysis and systems design methods, database management and data standards through interfaced information systems.

    a. True
    b. False

Match the terms in the left column with the correct descriptor in the right column. Not all descriptors may have an answer.

_____ 6. decision support system

_____ 7. computer-based patient record

_____ 8. local area network

_____ 9. data dictionary

_____ 10. database

_____ 11. data type

_____ 12. results reporting

a. text, numbers, voice and signals are examples

b. contains definitions for all the entities, attributes and relationships for data elements

c. system that is organized to receive clinical data from transaction systems and combine it with other data

d. a program that records access and/or action in a computer record by logging user information

e. a system which combines data with analysis tools to perform "what if" questions

f. an application designed to retrieve diagnostic and treatment results from feeder systems

g. data stored in fields, records and files

h. an electronic document on an individual that resides in a system

i. connects multiple devices via communications in a geographic area

13. Standard communication protocols are required of interfaced information systems.

    a. True
    b. False

14. A principal disadvantage of integrated information systems is that only departmental employees are authorized to change data.

    a. True
    b. False

15. What kind of health information system meets the needs of users external to the individual organization such as payers, researchers and planners?

    a. community health information system
    b. distributed health information system
    c. executive information system
    d. integrated health information system

16. The R-ADT system is a transaction oriented information system.

    a. True
    b. False

17. A point-of-care system is a documentation oriented information system.

    a. True
    b. False

18. A comprehensive health information system is comprised of:

    a. business and financial systems
    b. clinical information systems
    c. departmental systems
    d. all of the above

19. The MPI is considered a documentation system.

    a. True
    b. False

20. _____ is the process of scanning documents into a computerized system.

21. A turnaround document generally includes a computer-generated summary such as a discharge data abstract.

    a. True
    b. False

22. Networks permit access to centralized databases but not distributed databases.

    a. True
    b. False

23. Sponsors of health information systems include those who authorize, fund and use the information system.

    a. True
    b. False

24. Transaction-oriented systems support basic operational activities, such as pharmacy.

    a. True
    b. False

25. Decision-support systems and executive information systems are transaction-oriented systems.

    a. True
    b. False

26. When data are combined with analysis tools, the result is called a:

    a. clinical information system
    b. database management system
    c. decision-support system
    d. transaction-oriented system

27. A _____ supplies information system components for specified objectives.

28. Persons who rely on computer systems to perform their job are called _____.

29. Which represents an external expert system in a health information system?

    a. medical informatics
    b. National Library of Medicine
    c. electronic mail
    d. both b and c
    e. all of the above

30. Data security can be facilitated by the use of audit trails and turnaround documents.

    a. True
    b. False

31. An example of a data standard is a data dictionary.

    a. True
    b. False

32. Data type, data element and data item express the same thing.

    a. True
    b. False

33. Patient data can be expressed in natural language or text but not in coded form.

    a. True
    b. False

34. Query language is a form of text processing.

    a. True
    b. False

35. Natural language text must rely on semantic systems for processing.

    a. True
    b. False

36. The IOM sponsors the Computer-Based Patient Record Institute.

    a. True
    b. False

37. The data structure for the CPR is an integrated distributed database.

    a. True
    b. False

38. Which of the following collects clinical data from diverse sources in an integrated manner and reorganizes it for storage?

    a. data dictionary
    b. data repository
    c. database management system
    d. local area network

39. Data input and data output devices include all of the following *except:*
    a. sensors
    b. pocket devices
    c. CD ROM
    d. CPU

40. Which is an optical disc?

    a. COM
    b. CD ROM
    c. PDA
    d. CRT

41. _____ is an optical disc which is recorded at the site of the user and cannot be erased and re-recorded.

42. Which is not a customary standard software tool for a health care PC workstation?

    a. Telemedicine
    b. electronic mail
    c. word processing
    d. database

43. A patient record contains selected data elements for non-clinical uses called _____ data.

44. Referring to the data in question #43, name one use of this kind of patient data.

45. A repository of health information about a single patient is called a _____ record.

46. Computerized patient records include the processing of :

    a. numbers
    b. videos
    c. images
    d. all of the above

47. MEDLINE is a clinical reference database.

    a. True
    b. False

48. The most widely used database model, which is used for registries, for example, is:

    a. Internet
    b. medical informatics
    c. relational
    d. standard query language

PRETEST REVIEW ANSWER KEY

Directions:

1. Correct your Pretest Review Answer Sheet with the answers below by placing a slash (Example: ⌗) through the incorrect question number with a pen or pencil of a contrasting color.

2. Record the correct answer to the right of your answer on your answer sheet.

3. Record the total correct on the Initial Performance Grid in section four of this review manual.

4. Calculate your performance rate and also record on the grid.

5. Promptly locate the correct answer for each question missed in the chapter of the textbook.

6. Proceed to the chapter review if your performance rate was 80% or higher, otherwise, return to the chapter for further study.

Answers to Pretest Review

1.	a	5.	b	9.	a
2.	b	6.	a	10.	b
3.	a	7.	b	11.	b
4.	a	8.	b	12.	a

CHAPTER REVIEW ANSWER KEY

Directions:

1. Correct your Chapter Review Answer Sheet with the answers below by placing a slash (Example: ⌗) through the incorrect question number with a pen or pencil of a contrasting color.

2. Record the correct answer to the right of your answer on your answer sheet.

3. Record the total correct on the Initial Performance Grid in section four of this review manual.

4. Calculate your performance rate and also record on the grid.

5. Promptly locate the correct answer for each question missed in the chapter of the textbook.

6. Proceed to the next assigned chapter in your study.

Answers to Chapter Review

1.	a	6.	e	11.	a
2.	b	7.	h	12.	f
3.	a	8.	i	13.	a
4.	d	9.	b	14.	b
5.	b	10.	g	15.	a

16.	a	28.	users	40.	b
17.	a	29.	d	41.	WORM
18.	d	30.	b	42.	a
19.	a	31.	a	43.	secondary
20.	imaging	32.	b	44.	(any one) billing; QA, UR, RM; medical & legal audits; regulations, or administration
21.	b	33.	b		
22.	b	34.	b		
23.	b	35.	a	45.	patient or primary patient record or CPR or PPR
24.	a	36.	b		
25.	b	37.	a	46.	d
26.	c	38.	b	47.	b
27.	vendor	39.	d	48.	c

INFORMATION SYSTEMS LIFE CYCLE

18

PRETEST REVIEW

Directions:

1. Tear out a Pretest Review Answer Sheet from the back of this review manual.

2. Read each question carefully before selecting an answer.

3. Write the correct or best answer on the answer sheet.

4. Answer all the questions, since there is no penalty for this pretest review.

5. Check your answers with the answer key located near the end of this chapter.

1. A group process used in the analysis and design of an information system is referred to as GDSS.

    a. True
    b. False

2. A central repository identifying all data in a system is a data store.

    a. True
    b. False

3. Maintenance is one of the usual stages of an Information Systems Life Cycle.

    a. True
    b. False

4. Evaluation is one of the usual stages of a Systems Development Life Cycle.

    a. True
    b. False

5. An entity-relationship diagram illustrates the design of an information system database.

    a. True
    b. False

6. CASE can be helpful in operating an information system.

    a. True
    b. False

7. Development costs are to discounted payback period as investments costs in present dollars are to payback period.

    a. True
    b. False

8. The first stage in the system design process is the logical systems design.

    a. True
    b. False

9. RFPs are requested of vendors when entertaining the acquisition or expansion of an information system.

    a. True
    b. False

10. RFPs must contain technical, training and implementation specifications.

    a. True
    b. False

11. Matrix tables and data flow diagrams are tools useful to the analysis phase in the Systems Design Life Cycle.

    a. True
    b. False

12. Variability in information systems life cycles can result in a phenomenon called discontinuity.

    a. True
    b. False

CHAPTER REVIEW

Directions:

1. Tear out a Chapter Review Answer Sheet from the back of this review manual.

2. Read each question carefully before selecting an answer.

3. Write the correct or best answer on the answer sheet.

4. Answer all the questions since there is no penalty in this chapter review.

5. Check your answers with the answer key located at the end of this Chapter Review.

1. The maturity phase of the General Systems Life Cycle is similar to which phase in the Information Systems Life Cycle?

    a. growth
    b. implementation
    c. operation and maintenance
    d. obsolescence

2. Both information systems and technology are subject to obsolescence.

    a. True
    b. False

3. The organization-wide information systems life cycle conceptualized by Nolan consisted of four stages in the life cycle.

    a. True
    b. False

4. The data administration life cycle in the organization-wide information systems life cycle emphasizes the information, and its associated technologies and management, as being critical to the survival of the organization.

    a. True
    b. False

5. Which of the following examples is *not* descriptive of information systems obsolescence?

    a. mechanical failures with output devices or processing components
    b. turnover in users
    c. system enhancements to optimize the performance of tasks
    d. failure to support strategic organization change

6. Which is *not* a tool for systems analysis?

    a. control chart
    b. action diagram
    c. process specifications
    d. data structure

7. A hierarchy chart is a decomposition diagram.

    a. True
    b. False

8. Which is irrelevant to a hierarchy chart?

    a. parent node
    b. sibling node
    c. relationships
    d. functional primitives

9. ERDs are essentially a data map.

    a. True
    b. False

10. What are data stores and data flows related to?

    a. data dictionaries
    b. data flow diagrams
    c. decision trees
    d. none of the above

11. A data dictionary is a data repository.

    a. True
    b. False

12. Patients are an example of external entities in an information system.

    a. True
    b. False

13. Which is *not* a use of data flow diagrams?

    a. breaking down and grouping of tasks
    b. tracking the movement of data through a system
    c. identifying transformations of data
    d. identifying data stores

Project:	Record Completion Review System
Label:	Daily Discharge List
Entry Type:	Data Flow
Description:	Daily list of patients discharged from the hospital
Alias:	None
Composition:	Daily Discharge List = currentdate + medrecno + ptlname + ptfname + ptmidinital + ptdob + admitdate + dischgdate
Locations:	Context- and first-level explosions; second-level explosion of Process 1, Record Catalog
	Data Flow → Daily Discharge List

14. Referring to the illustration above, in what component of an information system would you find this notation?

15. Referring to the illustration at the top of the following page, what is the name of this diagram?

16. Referring to the illustration at the top of the following page, what is the appropriate name given the information depicted: *Admitting Department*?

17. Referring to the illustration at the top of the following page, what is the appropriate name given the information depicted: *Record Completion Review*?

18. Referring to the illustration at the top of the following page, what is the appropriate name given the information depicted: *permanent files*?

19. CASE is useful in the construction of the:

    a. entity-relationship diagram
    b. data flow diagram
    c. data dictionary
    d. all of the above

20. The length of a data element should be specified in the database.

    a. True
    b. False

21. Information about the process of a data element can be found in each of the following *except* the:

    a. explosion diagram
    b. data flow diagram
    c. data dictionary
    d. entity-relationship diagram

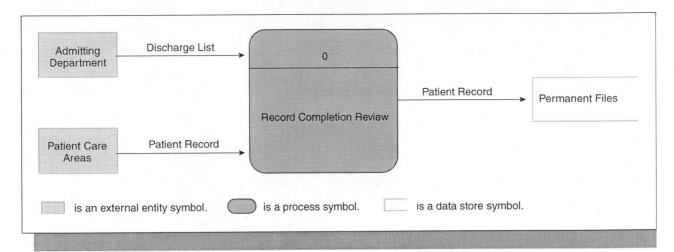

22. Information about entities can be found in each of the following *except* the:

    a. data dictionary
    b. entity-relationship diagram
    c. decomposition diagram
    d. data flow diagram

23. This symbol (⬜) is used in the construction of which tool?

    a. data dictionary
    b. entity-relationship diagram
    c. hierarchy chart
    d. data flow diagram

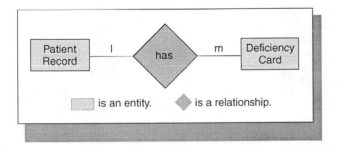

24. Referring to the illustration immediately above, what is the name of this diagram?

25. Referring to the illustration immediately above, "<u>m</u>" means what?

26. Referring to the illustration at the top of the following page, what name is given to the information underscored in the diagram: *patient record number and MDNO?*

27. Referring to the illustration at the top of the following page, "*1*" means what?

28. Which is descriptive of a data dictionary?

    a. specifies the data structures and data elements
    b. describes where data originate
    c. identifies data received by an area
    d. all of the above

29. Hierarchy charts are useful in the construction of explosion diagrams.

    a. True
    b. False

30. Transformations of data are processes and can be accurately depicted using this symbol: ⬜

    a. True
    b. False

31. Numbers are used in explosion diagrams to identify a process.

    a. True
    b. False

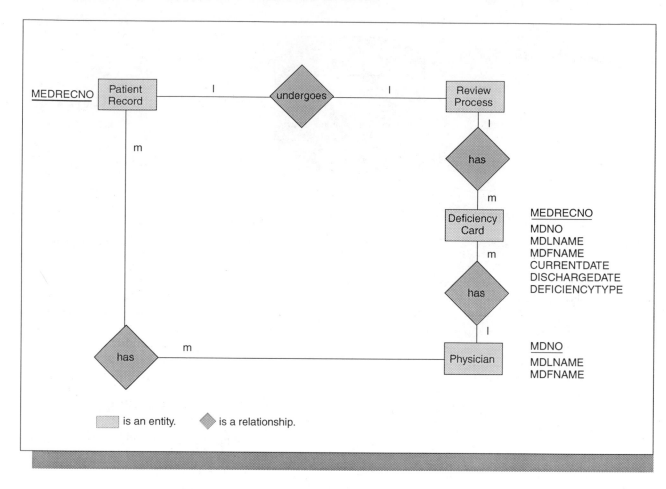

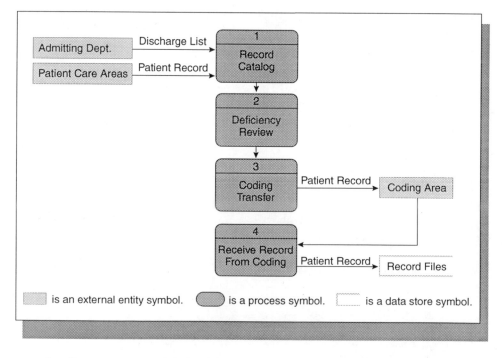

32. Referring to the illustration immediately above, what is the name for this diagram?

33. Referring to the illustration immediately above, what information depicts the level?

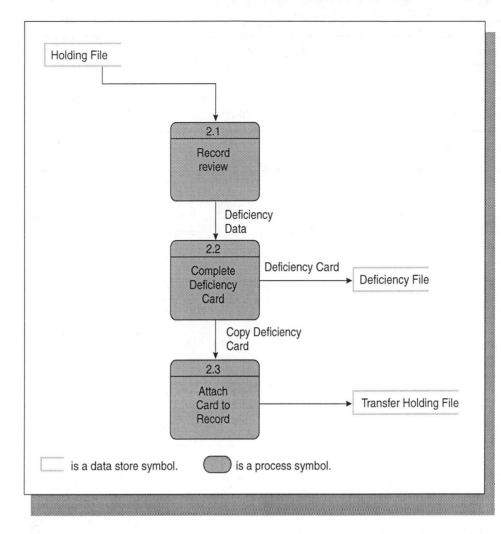

34. Referring to the illustration immediately above, what is the name for this diagram?

35. Referring to the information in the illustration, what process is depicted?

36. Where is the central repository for all information about a database maintained?

    a.   data dictionary
    b.   data structure
    c.   data store
    d.   all of the above

37. A data dictionary typically includes each of the following *except*:

    a.   range, values and meanings for data elements
    b.   data relationships
    c.   data flows
    d.   data stores

38. Explosions are used in conjunction with DFDs to depict the successive breakdown of a process.

    a.   True
    b.   False

39. Which of the following tools is used for the information system design of a database?

    a.   CASE
    b.   GDSS
    c.   entity-relationship diagram
    d.   interviews

	Year 1	Year 2	Year 3
Current System Cost	16,000	16,000	16,000
New System Cost	26,000	11,000	11,000
Yearly Difference in Costs	-10,000	+5,000	+5,000
Cumulative Difference in Costs			

40. Referring to the information in the table above, calculate the cumulative difference in costs. In which year will the payback period be reached?

  a. year 1
  b. year 2
  c. year 3
  d. none of the above

41. The phases of analysis, design, and implementation are collectively referred to as the:

  a. Information Systems Life Cycle
  b. System Development Life Cycle
  c. General System Life Cycle
  d. Strategic Plan

42. Which of the following is *not* a benefit of CASE tools?

  a. decreases development time
  b. increases standardization
  c. reduces errors
  d. lowers cost

43. Which of the following is true regarding the observation method for gathering data?

  a. It is less time consuming than questionnaire development.
  b. It is used to confirm or expand upon data collected from interviews.
  c. Little skill is required to conduct an observation.
  d. It is a non-obtrusive method for data gathering.

44. Which of the following is *not* a goal of an input process?

  a. make data input easy
  b. integrate the input process into regular work flow
  c. reduce duplication
  d. reduce efficiency

45. Which of the following is conducted to determine how well new program modules interact and execute with each other?

  a. unit testing
  b. system testing
  c. volume testing
  d. integration testing

46. Which of the following is *not* true about the benefits-realization process?

  a. It is economic-based.
  b. Criteria for evaluation are established before system installation.
  c. Measurements must be established for each evaluation criterion.
  d. Benefits are not measured compared to an economic outcome.

47. Which of the following could be included in the enterprise profile section of the RFP?

  a. functional specifications of the system
  b. technical requirements of the system
  c. overview of current departmental operations
  d. scenario-based problems with current system

48. Which of the following questions would be considered an unstructured question?

  a. Do you receive your computer reports on a daily basis?
  b. Do you have more than five microcomputers in your department?
  c. How many full-time-equivalent employees are in your department?
  d. How can the information systems department increase user satisfaction?

PRETEST REVIEW ANSWER KEY

Directions

1. Correct your Pretest Review Answer Sheet with the answers below by placing a slash (Example: 8) through the incorrect question number with a pen or pencil of a contrasting color.

2. Record the correct answer to the right of your answer on your answer sheet.

3. Record the total correct on the Initial Performance Grid in section four of this review manual.

4. Calculate your performance rate and also record on the grid.

5. Promptly locate the correct answer for each question missed in the chapter of the textbook.

6. Proceed to the chapter review if your performance rate was 80% or higher, otherwise, return to the chapter for further study.

1.	b	5.	a	9.	b
2.	b	6.	b	10.	a
3.	a	7.	b	11.	a
4.	b	8.	a	12.	a

CHAPTER REVIEW ANSWER KEY

Directions

1. Correct your Chapter Review Answer Sheet with the answers below by placing a slash (Example: 8) through the incorrect question number with a pen or pencil of a contrasting color.

2. Record the correct answer to the right of your answer on your answer sheet.

3. Record the total correct on the Initial Performance Grid in section four of this review manual.

4. Calculate your performance rate and also record on the grid.

5. Promptly locate the correct answer for each question missed in the chapter of the textbook.

6. Proceed to the next assigned chapter in your study.

1.	c	6.	a	11.	b
2.	a	7.	a	12.	a
3.	b	8.	c	13.	a
4.	a	9.	b	14.	data dictionary
5.	b	10.	b	15.	data flow diagramm or DFD

16. entity

17. process

18. data store

19. d

20. b

21. d

22. c

23. d

24. entity relationship diagram

25. many

26. key attributes

27. the patient record undergoes one review process

28. a

29. a

30. b

31. a

32. explosion diagram—first level explosion

33. whole number(s): # 1–4

34. second level explosion

35. process two

36. a

37. b

38. a

39. b

40. c

41. b

42. d

43. b

44. d

45. b

46. a

47. c

48. d

SECTION THREE

How to Prepare for Certification

INTRODUCTION AND APPLICATION

Certification is a process of testing a graduate's entry-level knowledge and competence in Health Information Management. The certification examinations for Medical Record Technicians (MRTs) and Medical Record Administrators (MRAs) are written by the American Health Information Management Association (AHIMA) and are administered by a testing agency once a year in the fall.

Successful passing of the respective examination certifies the graduate for practice at the entry level throughout the United States, Canada and Puerto Rico. This entrance level is described in the *Domains, Tasks and Subtasks*, published by AHIMA and included in section one of this review manual. Successful completion of the respective examination authorizes an individual to use the initials ART or RRA following his or her name. This credential can be retained and used as designated so long as the individual satisfies specified continuing education requirements of AHIMA.

Each certification examination can be taken in any one of 46 testing sites located throughout the United States and Puerto Rico and by special arrangement at other sites in or outside of the United States. These sites may cahnge from year-to-year.

Testing Center Sites

State	City	State	City	State	City
AK	Anchorage	MA	Boston	OK	Oklahoma City
AL	Birmingham	MD	Baltimore	OR	Portland
AR	Little Rock	ME	Bangor	PA	Philadelphia
AZ	Tempe	MI	Ann Arbor	PA	Pittsburgh
CA	Los Angeles	MN	Minneapolis	PR	Rio Piedras
CA	San Francisco	MO	Kansas City	SC	Columbia
CO	Denver	MO	St. Louis	SD	Sioux Falls
CT	New Haven	MS	Jackson	TN	Nashville
FL	Miami	MT	Great Falls	TX	Dallas
FL	Tampa	NC	Charlotte	TX	Houston
GA	Atlanta	ND	Fargo	TX	San Antonio
IA	Iowa City	NE	Omaha	UT	Salt Lake City
ID	Boise	NH	Concord	VA	Richmond
IL	Chicago	NM	Albuquerque	WA	Seattle
IN	Indianapolis	NY	New York	WI	Milwaukee
Ky	Louisville	NY	Syracuse	WV	Huntington
LA	Baton Rouge	OH	Columbus		

Each graduate makes application to write the respective examination for which he or she is a graduate. Application can be made after graduation by writing to the address below. Some college and university programs may provide applications for their graduates.

Applied Measurement Professionals
Attention: AHIMA Coordinator
8310 Nieman Road
Lenexa, KS 66214
(913) 541-0400

Certification Guide Contents

All applicants will receive a Certification Guide which provides detailed information about the examination:

Calendar of Examination Activities
General Examination Information
The Application Procedure
Test Administration
Examination Results and Scoring
Maintenance of Certification Requirements
Examination Content Outline
Sample Questions

CERTIFICATION EXAMINATION CONTENT

Each examination consists of multiple-choice questions requiring only one correct answer. Each examination measures the recall of knowledge, the application of knowledge and the resolution of problems.

- Knowledge and Comprehension Questions—This involves the recall of a wide range of material from specific facts to complete theories. It may involve translating material from one form to another (words to numbers), by interpreting material, and by predicting consequences or effects.

- Application Questions—This may include the application of such things as rules, methods, concepts, principles, laws, formulas, theories and standards.

- Analysis and Problem Solving Questions—This may include the interpretation of information, determining appropriate courses of action, and recognizing relationships.

The examinations are in two parts:

	MRA Exam	MRT Exam
Part I: HIM Competencies		
1. Questions	235	165
2. Time	3 hours + 45 minutes	2 hours + 30 minutes
Part II: Coding Competencies		
1. Questions	15	35
2. Time	45 minutes	1 hour + 45 minutes
TOTAL (Part I & II)		
1. Questions	250	200
2. Time	4 hours + 30 minutes	4 hours + 15 minutes

CERTIFICATION EXAMINATION COST

The application fee for both the Accreditation and Registration Examination may change from year-to-year. A fee of approximately $150 should be expected which can be payable by check, money order or VISA/MasterCard.

CERTIFICATION EXAMINATION SCORING

Each examination uses a standard answer sheet like the one shown on the following page. The examinations are machine scored by the testing agency giving equal weight to all the test questions. Although each examination has two sections, passing or failing is determined from the total number of correct responses on the entire examination.

Examinees receive their test results between eight and ten weeks following the examination. Approved applicants may retake the examination, as often as they wish to make application, until they achieve a passing score.

PREPARING FOR CERTIFICATION— BEFORE THE EXAM

- Begin your review well in advance of the examination. You might review your texts and classroom materials first, then practice by re-examining yourself on all chapters (by retaking all Pretests and Chapter Review tests using the extra answer sheets provided in the back). Or, you may wish to take each review test first, then use your notes and references for further study.

UAB

The University of Alabama at Birmingham
University of Alabama School of Medicine

NAME OF TEST

DATE OF TEST

CODES

LAST NAME

F.I. M.I.

SOCIAL SECURITY NO.

IMPORTANT

USE NO. 2 PENCIL ONLY

- EXAMPLE:
- ERASE *COMPLETELY* TO CHANGE
- INCORRECT MARKS

SCANTRON® FORM NO. F-1299-UAB   © SCANTRON CORPORATION 1990 ALL RIGHTS RESERVED.   2890-C871-5 4 3

- Avoid looking at the answers in the Answer Keys while completing each set of review questions.
- Leave items you cannot answer until you have completed both sets of questions. Then go back and try to answer those left blank. Sometimes other questions will provide clues or information essential for answering a question correctly that you have skipped.
- Read questions and possible answers carefully. Look for key words, such as "always," "never," "all," "except," "least," "best," and "not."
- Do not look for clues to correct answers such as a pattern , or a length of a response, for these are invalid and/or are controlled for in test construction.
- Know the location of your scheduled testing site. This information is provided by the testing agency a few weeks before the examination. If possible, it would be wise to make the trip to the site so that you can become familiar with the route and driving conditions (traffic). Locate the exact building, room and bathroom. Pay particular attention to parking locations and parking rules and to how long it took you to drive to the required location.
- Reread "Section One" of this Review Manual—*Helpful Test-Taking Principles* and your *Certification Guide—Test Administration*. The former will refresh your memory about test taking and the latter will remind you what you *must* take to the testing site for admittance.

- Eat a high protein, low fat breakfast before leaving for the testing site. You will not be given a lunch break; the total test time goes through the lunch hour. A high carbohydrate breakfast generally makes you hungry early (possibly hypoglycemic); a high fat breakfast may make you drowsy.

PREPARING FOR CERTIFICATION— DURING THE EXAM

- Do not burden yourself by taking books and papers into the testing site because they are not allowed in the examination room, except for coding books.
- Listen carefully to the examination directions given by the test proctor; read carefully the written instructions on the test book when distributed. Be clear when you can proceed to Part II of the examination.
- Skip and mark questions in both the test booklet and on the answer sheet that you want to return to. If time permits, return to those questions. It is better to guess than to leave an item blank.
- Do not be distracted by how fast others around you may be performing. Concentrate on your own performance and use of time.
- Review your work on the answer sheet carefully before submitting to the test proctor. Are all responses filled in neatly and darkly? Are all corrections *completely* erased? Are any items *unanswered*?

SECTION FOUR

How to Interpret Your Examination Readiness

This section includes three performance grids:

- The **Initial Performance Grid** to use upon chapter-by-chapter completion of this review manual.

- Repeat Performance Grids for two subsequent reviews, one for, perhaps, a final examination, and one for certification examination review after graduation.

- **Overall Performance Grid.** Once you have completed this manual and have filled in data on your performance grid, you can graph your performance for a visual display of your overall competence assessment. Upon doing this, notice in the example below, your performance can be displayed against a "standard" or "goal" which you can determine for yourself:

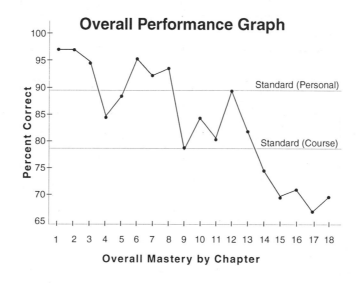

Overall Performance Graph

Overall Mastery by Chapter

In the above example, a male student set a personal goal of 90% to aim at in striving for mastery of the content. In addition to setting a personal standard, the student drew a horizontal line at 78% denoting what the course standard was for "passing" performance.

Then the student transferred each of the overall mastery percentages from Column 7 in the performance grid to the graph and connected them with straight lines.

Upon self-assessment of his performance against the standards, the student saw that he was successful in achieving "passing" performance in his review work on all the chapters except the last five. He attributed his performance on some of the first chapters in the book to their less complex content and decided that, other than a quick overview of that material, no extra effort or time was needed there.

The student considered, but eliminated, the notion that outside classroom activities could not be attributed to his low performance on Chapters 14-18. He attributed his performance solely to the level of difficulty of the material and to the more complex theory that went with the subject matter of the chapters. He decided he needed to do additional exercises in those subjects and to re-read the chapters more than once, plus complete some outside

recommended reading. He planned to retake the Chapter Reviews after re-reading the chapters and his notes until he achieved his personal goal of 90% on each one. While doing this, he was going to concentrate harder in understanding the underlying principles and reasons for the answers. He planned to use his initial performance graph to display his performance, except that he planned to do it in different colors of ink so that he could more easily analyze his repeated performance against his initial performance.

This student also reminded himself of the context the review manual played in his preparation. He remembered that the questions are few and merely a sampling of the total content. He decided, correctly, that the information in the graph was simply one index of his growing mastery and that he should not be solely dependent on its ability to translate into actual performance on the examination. He decided to add Chapters 9, 10, 11 and 13 to his review study program.

Until he wrote the unit exams, the student already expected that his adjustment in preparation would have to be repeated for the certifying examination if he wanted to increase his chances of passing and increase his personal confidence for that purpose.

	1	2	3	4	5	6	7
		# Pretest			# Chapter		% Overall Mastery
	# Pretest	Questions	% Pretest	# Chapter	Questions	% Chapter	$\frac{(col\ 2 + col\ 5)}{60}$
Chapter	Questions	Correct	Correct	Questions	Correct	Correct	
1	12			48			
2	12			48			
3	12			48			
4	12			48			
5	12			48			
6	12			48			
7	12			48			
8	12			48			
9	12			48			
10	12			48			
11	12			48			
12	12			48			
13	12			48			
14	12			48			
15	12			48			
16	12			48			
17	12			48			
18	12			48			
TOTAL	216			864			

INITIAL PERFORMANCE GRID

REPEAT PERFORMANCE GRID

Chapter	1 # Pretest Questions	2 # Pretest Questions Correct	3 % Pretest Correct	4 # Chapter Questions	5 # Chapter Questions Correct	6 % Chapter Correct	7 % Overall Mastery (col 2 + col 5)/60
1	12			48			
2	12			48			
3	12			48			
4	12			48			
5	12			48			
6	12			48			
7	12			48			
8	12			48			
9	12			48			
10	12			48			
11	12			48			
12	12			48			
13	12			48			
14	12			48			
15	12			48			
16	12			48			
17	12			48			
18	12			48			
TOTAL	216			864			

REPEAT PERFORMANCE GRID

Chapter	1 # Pretest Questions	2 # Pretest Questions Correct	3 % Pretest Correct	4 # Chapter Questions	5 # Chapter Questions Correct	6 % Chapter Correct	7 % Overall Mastery $\frac{(col\ 2 + col\ 5)}{60}$
1	12			48			
2	12			48			
3	12			48			
4	12			48			
5	12			48			
6	12			48			
7	12			48			
8	12			48			
9	12			48			
10	12			48			
11	12			48			
12	12			48			
13	12			48			
14	12			48			
15	12			48			
16	12			48			
17	12			48			
18	12			48			
TOTAL	216			864			

PRETEST REVIEW—ANSWER SHEET

Chapter Number _____

Chapter Title_____

1. _____   7. _____

2. _____   8. _____

3. _____   9. _____

4. _____   10. _____

5. _____   11. _____

6. _____   12. _____

Proceed to the Performance Grid. Return to the textbook to review the material for questions not answered correctly. Proceed to the Chapter Review.

PRETEST REVIEW—ANSWER SHEET

Chapter Number _____

Chapter Title_____

1. _____   7. _____

2. _____   8. _____

3. _____   9. _____

4. _____   10. _____

5. _____   11. _____

6. _____   12. _____

Proceed to the Performance Grid. Return to the textbook to review the material for questions not answered correctly. Proceed to the Chapter Review.

PRETEST REVIEW—ANSWER SHEET

Chapter Number _____

Chapter Title_____

1. _____   7. _____

2. _____   8. _____

3. _____   9. _____

4. _____   10. _____

5. _____   11. _____

6. _____   12. _____

Proceed to the Performance Grid. Return to the textbook to review the material for questions not answered correctly. Proceed to the Chapter Review.

PRETEST REVIEW—ANSWER SHEET

Chapter Number _____

Chapter Title_____

1. _____   7. _____

2. _____   8. _____

3. _____   9. _____

4. _____   10. _____

5. _____   11. _____

6. _____   12. _____

Proceed to the Performance Grid. Return to the textbook to review the material for questions not answered correctly. Proceed to the Chapter Review.

PRETEST REVIEW—ANSWER SHEET

Chapter Number _____

Chapter Title_____

1. _____   7. _____

2. _____   8. _____

3. _____   9. _____

4. _____   10. _____

5. _____   11. _____

6. _____   12. _____

Proceed to the Performance Grid. Return to the textbook to review the material for questions not answered correctly. Proceed to the Chapter Review.

PRETEST REVIEW—ANSWER SHEET

Chapter Number _____

Chapter Title_____

1. _____   7. _____

2. _____   8. _____

3. _____   9. _____

4. _____   10. _____

5. _____   11. _____

6. _____   12. _____

Proceed to the Performance Grid. Return to the textbook to review the material for questions not answered correctly. Proceed to the Chapter Review.

PRETEST REVIEW—ANSWER SHEET

Chapter Number _____

Chapter Title_____

1. _____

2. _____

3. _____

4. _____

5. _____

6. _____

7. _____

8. _____

9. _____

10. _____

11. _____

12. _____

Proceed to the Performance Grid. Return to the textbook to review the material for questions not answered correctly. Proceed to the Chapter Review.

PRETEST REVIEW—ANSWER SHEET

Chapter Number _____

Chapter Title_____

1. _____   7. _____

2. _____   8. _____

3. _____   9. _____

4. _____   10. _____

5. _____   11. _____

6. _____   12. _____

Proceed to the Performance Grid. Return to the textbook to review the material for questions not answered correctly. Proceed to the Chapter Review.

PRETEST REVIEW—ANSWER SHEET

Chapter Number _____

Chapter Title_____

1. _____

2. _____

3. _____

4. _____

5. _____

6. _____

7. _____

8. _____

9. _____

10. _____

11. _____

12. _____

Proceed to the Performance Grid. Return to the textbook to review the material for questions not answered correctly. Proceed to the Chapter Review.

PRETEST REVIEW—ANSWER SHEET

Chapter Number _____

Chapter Title_____

1. _____   7. _____

2. _____   8. _____

3. _____   9. _____

4. _____   10. _____

5. _____   11. _____

6. _____   12. _____

Proceed to the Performance Grid. Return to the textbook to review the material for questions not answered correctly. Proceed to the Chapter Review.

PRETEST REVIEW—ANSWER SHEET

Chapter Number _____

Chapter Title_____

1. _____   7. _____

2. _____   8. _____

3. _____   9. _____

4. _____   10. _____

5. _____   11. _____

6. _____   12. _____

Proceed to the Performance Grid. Return to the textbook to review the material for questions not answered correctly. Proceed to the Chapter Review.

PRETEST REVIEW—ANSWER SHEET

Chapter Number _____

Chapter Title _____

1. _____   7. _____

2. _____   8. _____

3. _____   9. _____

4. _____   10. _____

5. _____   11. _____

6. _____   12. _____

Proceed to the Performance Grid. Return to the textbook to review the material for questions not answered correctly. Proceed to the Chapter Review.

PRETEST REVIEW—ANSWER SHEET

Chapter Number _____

Chapter Title_____

1. _____   7. _____

2. _____   8. _____

3. _____   9. _____

4. _____   10. _____

5. _____   11. _____

6. _____   12. _____

Proceed to the Performance Grid. Return to the textbook to review the material for questions not answered correctly. Proceed to the Chapter Review.

PRETEST REVIEW—ANSWER SHEET

Chapter Number _____

Chapter Title_____

1. _____   7. _____

2. _____   8. _____

3. _____   9. _____

4. _____   10. _____

5. _____   11. _____

6. _____   12. _____

Proceed to the Performance Grid. Return to the textbook to review the material for questions not answered correctly. Proceed to the Chapter Review.

PRETEST REVIEW—ANSWER SHEET

Chapter Number _____

Chapter Title_____

1. _____   7. _____

2. _____   8. _____

3. _____   9. _____

4. _____   10. _____

5. _____   11. _____

6. _____   12. _____

Proceed to the Performance Grid. Return to the textbook to review the material for questions not answered correctly. Proceed to the Chapter Review.

PRETEST REVIEW—ANSWER SHEET

Chapter Number _____

Chapter Title_____

1. _____   7. _____

2. _____   8. _____

3. _____   9. _____

4. _____   10. _____

5. _____   11. _____

6. _____   12. _____

Proceed to the Performance Grid. Return to the textbook to review the material for questions not answered correctly. Proceed to the Chapter Review.

PRETEST REVIEW—ANSWER SHEET

Chapter Number _____

Chapter Title_____

1. _____   7. _____

2. _____   8. _____

3. _____   9. _____

4. _____   10. _____

5. _____   11. _____

6. _____   12. _____

Proceed to the Performance Grid. Return to the textbook to review the material for questions not answered correctly. Proceed to the Chapter Review.

PRETEST REVIEW—ANSWER SHEET

Chapter Number _____

Chapter Title_____

1. _____   7. _____

2. _____   8. _____

3. _____   9. _____

4. _____   10. _____

5. _____   11. _____

6. _____   12. _____

Proceed to the Performance Grid. Return to the textbook to review the material for questions not answered correctly. Proceed to the Chapter Review.

CHAPTER REVIEW—ANSWER SHEET

Chapter Number _____

Chapter Title_____

1 . _____	25. _____
2. _____	26. _____
3. _____	27. _____
4. _____	28. _____
5. _____	29 . _____
6. _____	30. _____
7. _____	31. _____
8. _____	32. _____
9. _____	33. _____
10. _____	34. _____
11. _____	35. _____
12. _____	36. _____
13. _____	37. _____
14. _____	38. _____
15. _____	39. _____
16. _____	40. _____
17. _____	41. _____
18. _____	42. _____
19. _____	43. _____
20. _____	44. _____
21. _____	45. _____
22. _____	46. _____
23. _____	47. _____
24. _____	48. _____

Proceed to the Performance Grid. Return to the textbook to review the material for questions not answered correctly.

CHAPTER REVIEW—ANSWER SHEET

Chapter Number _____

Chapter Title_____

1 . _____	25. _____
2. _____	26. _____
3. _____	27. _____
4. _____	28. _____
5. _____	29 . _____
6. _____	30. _____
7. _____	31. _____
8. _____	32. _____
9. _____	33. _____
10. _____	34. _____
11. _____	35. _____
12. _____	36. _____
13. _____	37. _____
14. _____	38. _____
15. _____	39. _____
16. _____	40. _____
17. _____	41. _____
18. _____	42. _____
19. _____	43. _____
20. _____	44. _____
21. _____	45. _____
22. _____	46. _____
23. _____	47. _____
24. _____	48. _____

Proceed to the Performance Grid. Return to the textbook to review the material for questions not answered correctly.

CHAPTER REVIEW—ANSWER SHEET

Chapter Number _____

Chapter Title_____

1 . _____	25. _____
2. _____	26. _____
3. _____	27. _____
4. _____	28. _____
5. _____	29 . _____
6. _____	30. _____
7. _____	31. _____
8. _____	32. _____
9. _____	33. _____
10. _____	34. _____
11. _____	35. _____
12. _____	36. _____
13. _____	37. _____
14. _____	38. _____
15. _____	39. _____
16. _____	40. _____
17. _____	41. _____
18. _____	42. _____
19. _____	43. _____
20. _____	44. _____
21. _____	45. _____
22. _____	46. _____
23. _____	47. _____
24. _____	48. _____

Proceed to the Performance Grid. Return to the textbook to review the material for questions not answered correctly.

CHAPTER REVIEW—ANSWER SHEET

Chapter Number _____

Chapter Title_____

1. _____	25. _____
2. _____	26. _____
3. _____	27. _____
4. _____	28. _____
5. _____	29. _____
6. _____	30. _____
7. _____	31. _____
8. _____	32. _____
9. _____	33. _____
10. _____	34. _____
11. _____	35. _____
12. _____	36. _____
13. _____	37. _____
14. _____	38. _____
15. _____	39. _____
16. _____	40. _____
17. _____	41. _____
18. _____	42. _____
19. _____	43. _____
20. _____	44. _____
21. _____	45. _____
22. _____	46. _____
23. _____	47. _____
24. _____	48. _____

Proceed to the Performance Grid. Return to the textbook to review the material for questions not answered correctly.

CHAPTER REVIEW—ANSWER SHEET

Chapter Number _____

Chapter Title _____

1. _____   25. _____
2. _____   26. _____
3. _____   27. _____
4. _____   28. _____
5. _____   29. _____
6. _____   30. _____
7. _____   31. _____
8. _____   32. _____
9. _____   33. _____
10. _____   34. _____
11. _____   35. _____
12. _____   36. _____
13. _____   37. _____
14. _____   38. _____
15. _____   39. _____
16. _____   40. _____
17. _____   41. _____
18. _____   42. _____
19. _____   43. _____
20. _____   44. _____
21. _____   45. _____
22. _____   46. _____
23. _____   47. _____
24. _____   48. _____

Proceed to the Performance Grid. Return to the textbook to review the material for questions not answered correctly.

CHAPTER REVIEW—ANSWER SHEET

Chapter Number _____

Chapter Title_____

1. _____	25. _____
2. _____	26. _____
3. _____	27. _____
4. _____	28. _____
5. _____	29. _____
6. _____	30. _____
7. _____	31. _____
8. _____	32. _____
9. _____	33. _____
10. _____	34. _____
11. _____	35. _____
12. _____	36. _____
13. _____	37. _____
14. _____	38. _____
15. _____	39. _____
16. _____	40. _____
17. _____	41. _____
18. _____	42. _____
19. _____	43. _____
20. _____	44. _____
21. _____	45. _____
22. _____	46. _____
23. _____	47. _____
24. _____	48. _____

Proceed to the Performance Grid. Return to the textbook to review the material for questions not answered correctly.

CHAPTER REVIEW—ANSWER SHEET

Chapter Number _____

Chapter Title_____

1 . _____	25. _____
2. _____	26. _____
3. _____	27. _____
4. _____	28. _____
5. _____	29 . _____
6. _____	30. _____
7. _____	31. _____
8. _____	32. _____
9. _____	33. _____
10. _____	34. _____
11. _____	35. _____
12. _____	36. _____
13. _____	37. _____
14. _____	38. _____
15. _____	39. _____
16. _____	40. _____
17. _____	41. _____
18. _____	42. _____
19. _____	43. _____
20. _____	44. _____
21. _____	45. _____
22. _____	46. _____
23. _____	47. _____
24. _____	48. _____

Proceed to the Performance Grid. Return to the textbook to review the material for questions not answered correctly.

CHAPTER REVIEW—ANSWER SHEET

Chapter Number _____

Chapter Title_____

1. _____	25. _____
2. _____	26. _____
3. _____	27. _____
4. _____	28. _____
5. _____	29. _____
6. _____	30. _____
7. _____	31. _____
8. _____	32. _____
9. _____	33. _____
10. _____	34. _____
11. _____	35. _____
12. _____	36. _____
13. _____	37. _____
14. _____	38. _____
15. _____	39. _____
16. _____	40. _____
17. _____	41. _____
18. _____	42. _____
19. _____	43. _____
20. _____	44. _____
21. _____	45. _____
22. _____	46. _____
23. _____	47. _____
24. _____	48. _____

Proceed to the Performance Grid. Return to the textbook to review the material for questions not answered correctly.

CHAPTER REVIEW—ANSWER SHEET

Chapter Number _____

Chapter Title_____

1. _____	25. _____
2. _____	26. _____
3. _____	27. _____
4. _____	28. _____
5. _____	29. _____
6. _____	30. _____
7. _____	31. _____
8. _____	32. _____
9. _____	33. _____
10. _____	34. _____
11. _____	35. _____
12. _____	36. _____
13. _____	37. _____
14. _____	38. _____
15. _____	39. _____
16. _____	40. _____
17. _____	41. _____
18. _____	42. _____
19. _____	43. _____
20. _____	44. _____
21. _____	45. _____
22. _____	46. _____
23. _____	47. _____
24. _____	48. _____

Proceed to the Performance Grid. Return to the textbook to review the material for questions not answered correctly.

CHAPTER REVIEW—ANSWER SHEET

Chapter Number _____

Chapter Title_____

1 . _____	25. _____
2. _____	26. _____
3. _____	27. _____
4. _____	28. _____
5. _____	29 . _____
6. _____	30. _____
7. _____	31. _____
8. _____	32. _____
9. _____	33. _____
10. _____	34. _____
11. _____	35. _____
12. _____	36. _____
13. _____	37. _____
14. _____	38. _____
15. _____	39. _____
16. _____	40. _____
17. _____	41. _____
18. _____	42. _____
19. _____	43. _____
20. _____	44. _____
21. _____	45. _____
22. _____	46. _____
23. _____	47. _____
24. _____	48. _____

Proceed to the Performance Grid. Return to the textbook to review the material for questions not answered correctly.

CHAPTER REVIEW—ANSWER SHEET

Chapter Number _____

Chapter Title_____

1 . _____	25. _____
2. _____	26. _____
3. _____	27. _____
4. _____	28. _____
5. _____	29 . _____
6. _____	30. _____
7. _____	31. _____
8. _____	32. _____
9. _____	33. _____
10. _____	34. _____
11. _____	35. _____
12. _____	36. _____
13. _____	37. _____
14. _____	38. _____
15. _____	39. _____
16. _____	40. _____
17. _____	41. _____
18. _____	42. _____
19. _____	43. _____
20. _____	44. _____
21. _____	45. _____
22. _____	46. _____
23. _____	47. _____
24. _____	48. _____

Proceed to the Performance Grid. Return to the textbook to review the material for questions not answered correctly.

CHAPTER REVIEW—ANSWER SHEET

Chapter Number _____

Chapter Title_____

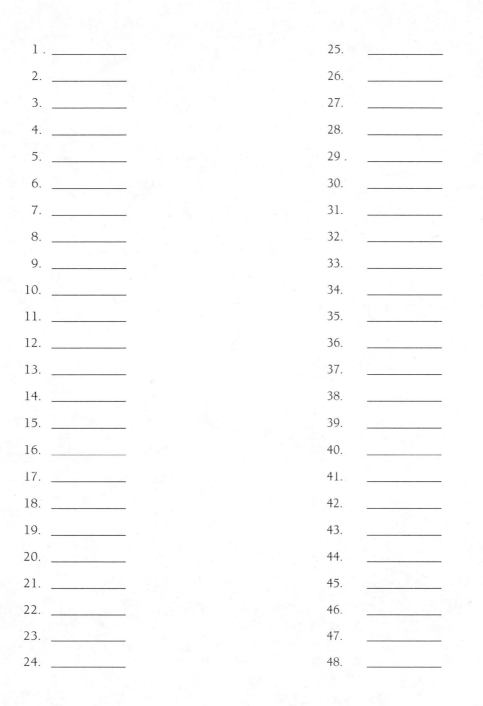

1. _____		25. _____	
2. _____		26. _____	
3. _____		27. _____	
4. _____		28. _____	
5. _____		29. _____	
6. _____		30. _____	
7. _____		31. _____	
8. _____		32. _____	
9. _____		33. _____	
10. _____		34. _____	
11. _____		35. _____	
12. _____		36. _____	
13. _____		37. _____	
14. _____		38. _____	
15. _____		39. _____	
16. _____		40. _____	
17. _____		41. _____	
18. _____		42. _____	
19. _____		43. _____	
20. _____		44. _____	
21. _____		45. _____	
22. _____		46. _____	
23. _____		47. _____	
24. _____		48. _____	

Proceed to the Performance Grid. Return to the textbook to review the material for questions not answered correctly.

CHAPTER REVIEW—ANSWER SHEET

Chapter Number _____

Chapter Title_____

1. _____	25. _____
2. _____	26. _____
3. _____	27. _____
4. _____	28. _____
5. _____	29. _____
6. _____	30. _____
7. _____	31. _____
8. _____	32. _____
9. _____	33. _____
10. _____	34. _____
11. _____	35. _____
12. _____	36. _____
13. _____	37. _____
14. _____	38. _____
15. _____	39. _____
16. _____	40. _____
17. _____	41. _____
18. _____	42. _____
19. _____	43. _____
20. _____	44. _____
21. _____	45. _____
22. _____	46. _____
23. _____	47. _____
24. _____	48. _____

Proceed to the Performance Grid. Return to the textbook to review the material for questions not answered correctly.

CHAPTER REVIEW—ANSWER SHEET

Chapter Number _____

Chapter Title_____

1. _____	25. _____
2. _____	26. _____
3. _____	27. _____
4. _____	28. _____
5. _____	29. _____
6. _____	30. _____
7. _____	31. _____
8. _____	32. _____
9. _____	33. _____
10. _____	34. _____
11. _____	35. _____
12. _____	36. _____
13. _____	37. _____
14. _____	38. _____
15. _____	39. _____
16. _____	40. _____
17. _____	41. _____
18. _____	42. _____
19. _____	43. _____
20. _____	44. _____
21. _____	45. _____
22. _____	46. _____
23. _____	47. _____
24. _____	48. _____

Proceed to the Performance Grid. Return to the textbook to review the material for questions not answered correctly.

CHAPTER REVIEW—ANSWER SHEET

Chapter Number _____

Chapter Title_____

1. _____	25. _____
2. _____	26. _____
3. _____	27. _____
4. _____	28. _____
5. _____	29. _____
6. _____	30. _____
7. _____	31. _____
8. _____	32. _____
9. _____	33. _____
10. _____	34. _____
11. _____	35. _____
12. _____	36. _____
13. _____	37. _____
14. _____	38. _____
15. _____	39. _____
16. _____	40. _____
17. _____	41. _____
18. _____	42. _____
19. _____	43. _____
20. _____	44. _____
21. _____	45. _____
22. _____	46. _____
23. _____	47. _____
24. _____	48. _____

Proceed to the Performance Grid. Return to the textbook to review the material for questions not answered correctly.

CHAPTER REVIEW—ANSWER SHEET

Chapter Number _____

Chapter Title_____

1 . _____			25. _____	
2. _____			26. _____	
3. _____			27. _____	
4. _____			28. _____	
5. _____			29 . _____	
6. _____			30. _____	
7. _____			31. _____	
8. _____			32. _____	
9. _____			33. _____	
10. _____			34. _____	
11. _____			35. _____	
12. _____			36. _____	
13. _____			37. _____	
14. _____			38. _____	
15. _____			39. _____	
16. _____			40. _____	
17. _____			41. _____	
18. _____			42. _____	
19. _____			43. _____	
20. _____			44. _____	
21. _____			45. _____	
22. _____			46. _____	
23. _____			47. _____	
24. _____			48. _____	

Proceed to the Performance Grid. Return to the textbook to review the material for questions not answered correctly.

CHAPTER REVIEW—ANSWER SHEET

Chapter Number _____

Chapter Title_____

1. _____	25. _____
2. _____	26. _____
3. _____	27. _____
4. _____	28. _____
5. _____	29. _____
6. _____	30. _____
7. _____	31. _____
8. _____	32. _____
9. _____	33. _____
10. _____	34. _____
11. _____	35. _____
12. _____	36. _____
13. _____	37. _____
14. _____	38. _____
15. _____	39. _____
16. _____	40. _____
17. _____	41. _____
18. _____	42. _____
19. _____	43. _____
20. _____	44. _____
21. _____	45. _____
22. _____	46. _____
23. _____	47. _____
24. _____	48. _____

Proceed to the Performance Grid. Return to the textbook to review the material for questions not answered correctly.

CHAPTER REVIEW—ANSWER SHEET

Chapter Number _____

Chapter Title_____

1. _____	25. _____
2. _____	26. _____
3. _____	27. _____
4. _____	28. _____
5. _____	29. _____
6. _____	30. _____
7. _____	31. _____
8. _____	32. _____
9. _____	33. _____
10. _____	34. _____
11. _____	35. _____
12. _____	36. _____
13. _____	37. _____
14. _____	38. _____
15. _____	39. _____
16. _____	40. _____
17. _____	41. _____
18. _____	42. _____
19. _____	43. _____
20. _____	44. _____
21. _____	45. _____
22. _____	46. _____
23. _____	47. _____
24. _____	48. _____

Proceed to the Performance Grid. Return to the textbook to review the material for questions not answered correctly.